This small volume was never intended to be a comprehensive work on the subject of poisoning. That would have made it far too massive to be compressed between these two slim covers. Rather is it a book designed as what used to be called a *vade-mecum*; that is, almost literally, a constant companion to which reference can immediately be made, hopefully with benefit. The critics are sure to discover omissions, for prominence has been given, first to common types of acute poisoning likely to be encountered in everyday clinical practice and, second, to the general principles of diagnosis and, more so, of management, adherence to which will afford a reasonably sensible, safe and helpful course of action, regardless of the specific nature of the toxic agent that has been involved.

The introductory section might be regarded as falling somewhat outside this plan. Just as with other diseases, though, poisoning is not a simple nosological entity; it must be viewed medically in its wider context. That is why the reader is invited, at the outset, to spend a few minutes on Chapter 1, just to put the practical aspect into perspective.

Thereafter, the immediate care of the patient demands attention, irrespective of the cause. Emergency measures for survival having been accomplished, thought must be given to the applicability of specific antidotes. Not that these will be appropriate in many instances, but, wherever they are indicated, they should be mobilised without delay. Subsequently and with forethought, the ongoing care, especially in the realm of intensive treatment, should be put into effect, bearing in mind then the assistance that can be offered by laboratory investigations.

Finally, thought should be given to the ultimate outcome and welfare of the patient, not overlooking the possible forensic implications.

No one, except he be arrogant, is master of every eventuality, even within the limited specialty of acute poisoning. The greater part of the content of this book has been based on personal experience. At the same time knowledge and advice from other sources, both textual and personal, has been unashamedly brought to bear on what has been written here. Without nominating individuals, for fear of invidiously disregarding someone who ought to have been mentioned, I would like to express my gratitude and appreciation all-embracingly for the immense help and inspiration that I have derived from my colleagues, over the years, in the Poisons Unit at Guy's Hospital, London.

It is also customary in a preface to acknowledge the assistance afforded by one's publishers. To do so on this occasion is far from specious. They have borne, with patience and fortitude, all my idiosyncracies and delays and, at the same time, offered valuable suggestions and guidance, the adoption of which can have done no other than improve the final version.

All of the figures have been derived from *Poisoning: Diagnosis and Treatment* (1981) edited by J.A. Vale and T.J. Meredith by kind permission of the editors and Update Books.

Roy Goulding

1.0 Introduction

Contents

615.9

GOU

0632010940

(28.5.97)

1.0 Introduction

1.1 Toxins: poisons

Colloquially, everyone knows what poisoning is. A substance is surreptitiously slipped into a person's food, or drink, and within a short time of swallowing it, the victim slumps down dead. But that is just acute poisoning, homicidally actuated. Today, more publicity, often sensational, is generated about poisons in the environment, with their supposed delayed and insidious evils. So it may be as well, at the outset, to set out a few explanations and definitions.

There are three indispensable components to the phenomenon of poisoning:

1 *The toxin* itself, i.e. a noxious substance.
2 *The subject*, or living system, to which it gains access.
3 *The adverse effects* which follow.

Without all of these three factors, poisoning cannot be said to have occurred.

1.1 Toxins: poisons

Statutorily, at least in the United Kingdom, a poison is not precisely defined, for instance under the Offences Against the Person Act (1861) it is taken to apply to any 'noxious thing' that may cause death, assist in the committing of an indictable offence, endanger life or inflict grievous bodily harm, burning, disfigurement, etc., injure, aggrieve or annoy. The description obviously caters for a wide range of possibilities, as sensibly it should. Almost any substance, of mineral, vegetable, animal, or synthetic origin, can in fact function as a poison, given a suitable dose and circumstances; however some materials are intrinsically more toxic than others. Thus, less than a gram of potassium cyanide taken by mouth is likely to bring about the death of a person in the course of minutes, while even less of the plant toxin, ricin, injected into a muscle, will prove fatal some days later. On the other hand, sodium chloride, which as culinary salt is habitually regarded as an article of diet, can be lethal if a large enough dose is given, above all if it is repeated. So it has become a convention to differentiate substances according to their inherent toxicity.

There is, however, no absolute measure of toxicity, for this is a biological and not a physical characteristic and so varies according to the species, age, sex, state of health, environmental conditions, route of administration, etc., applying to the subject. The concept has nevertheless been adopted of referring to the lethal dose of a substance, expressed in terms of milligrams per kilogram body weight, but even then it is imperative to name at least the species, the sex and the route of administration. Moreover, to bring some uniformity to natural variation, what is called the median lethal dose (MLD) may be arrived at mathematically from experiments on different groups of animals, each given a different dose level, with the outcome being measured as numbers being killed. In this manner, descriptively speaking, the MLD represents that amount of the substance (as mg kg^{-1} body weight) that would, by this calculation, kill 50% of these animals.

1.2 The subject

From the biological standpoint, no poison is dangerous in itself as, say, when it is stored in a secure container. For its toxicity to be evoked it must gain entry into a living system by one means or another, via the mouth, the breath, through the skin or by some other route. This may appear self-evident, but in clinical practice poisoning can be veritably diagnosed only if uptake by the tissues can be confirmed. Mere propinquity is enough to suggest only **suspected poisoning.**

1.3 Adverse effects

These may be minor or serious, transient or permanent, or even fatal, but they must be manifest for poisoning to be declared. A drug such as phenobarbitone, given in the correct dose to suppress epilepsy, is a prophylactic agent, with a beneficial influence, but when the identical medicament is taken in an overdose such that it imperils respiration and consciousness and ultimately causes death, then it is a poison.

1.4 Modes of exposure

A common route of administration is the **oral** one. The consequences then will depend on the extent to which absorption takes place from the gastrointestinal tract. Metallic mercury, for example, does not find its way readily through the alimentary mucosa and, given by mouth, is seldom dangerous; mercurous iodide is similar. By contrast, ethyl mercuric salts given in this way may be pronouncedly toxic because they are then readily taken up systemically.

Some toxins can be **inhaled**. Metallic mercury is quick to volatilise into the atmosphere, and in this way it may be taken in with the breath to produce deleterious effects. Similarly, arsine, phosgene and chlorine may be devastating by the respiratory route.

The **skin**, moreover, is not a totally impervious barrier. Again, metallic mercury in repeated contact with the skin, as in the old-fashioned manner of treating syphilis, or as happened when it was incorporated into finger-printing powders, or as an ingredient of certain ethnic cosmetics, may penetrate the tissues in systemically poisonous concentrations.

Clearly, the **injection** of substances into the body brings them into close relationship with the circulation and thus the organs. Ricin has already been mentioned in this respect. An excess of thiopentone intravenously can provoke acute laryngospasm, as well as central nervous system depression, while halothane, otherwise an acceptable inhalation anaesthetic, can be lethal when inadvertently introduced into the veins.

Even the **rectal** route has its risks. Overdoses have been recorded from drugs such as tribromoethanol and paraldehyde given injudiciously in this way. The **vagina**, too, can provide for systemic entry, an excess of acetarsol suppositories having set up catastrophic arsenical poisoning.

1.5 Species variation

Not all animals respond identically to the same agent. In the guinea-pig, penicillin by injection can be disastrous; in man it is almost innocuous—apart from sensitisation reactions. The rat, lacking the capacity to vomit, is overcome by squills given orally, whereas the dog, able to vomit easily, is virtually immune to this rodenticide. For this reason it is both naive and unwise to assume that all species are toxicologically identical and, more so, to extrapolate directly and unreservedly from animal to man.

1.6   Individual variation

A collection of even one species is not a biologically homo-
geneous population. Individuals react differently to the same
noxious stimulus. de Quincey, for one, could take inordinate
libations of opium which would have killed another person.
Admittedly he had built up **tolerance**, whereby the habitual
dosing of a drug results in it becoming inefficacious in the
customary doses and progressively increased amounts have to be
taken to achieve any effect. Rasputin, too, is reputed to have
been unscathed by a dose of cyanide that would have felled
another man. Over recent years, moreover, the need to 'tailor'
therapeutic doses of drugs to bring about the same response in
different patients has become impressive.

The object of the foregoing paragraphs has been to emphasise
that, in clinical toxicology, just as in other medical specialities, no
universal formula can be applied. Glib assumptions have no place
in practice and each patient must be assessed on the individual
merits and treated accordingly.

1.7   Types of poisoning

Acute poisoning, with one dose, or one exposure, being
succeeded shortly by an associated response, is probably the
simplest toxic phenomenon. But poisoning can also be brought
about over the **short-term**, with repeated doses or exposures,
each in itself inconsequential, culminating in a delayed effect,
usually on account of **cumulation** that leads to an overwhelming
body burden. This is seen in chronic lead poisoning. Still more
delayed is the mechanism of carcinogenesis, when protracted
contact with, for example, arsenic, vinyl chloride monomer,
asbestos, benzidine, cigarette smoke, etc., can predispose to
neoplasia decades later, without necessarily any cumulation of the
causal agent in the body.

In the clinical arena, therefore, poisoning can present in a variety
of forms. For the purpose of this text, however, priority will be
given to acute poisoning, for it is on this account that the aid of
the physician is most commonly summoned. Food poisoning,
though it cannot be disregarded by the doctor, is of microbiological origin and, being aetiologically so distinct, will not be
included herein.

1.8 Causation

Poisoning may come about *accidentally*, or *intentionally*. With adults, something may be taken by mistake, or exposure may beset someone unwittingly, at work, or in the environment. Small children are prone deliberately, albeit innocently, to put toxic things into their mouths. These events are all regarded as accidental.

Quite distinct are those acts in which someone premeditatively sets out to poison someone else, i.e. **homicide**. Much more common nowadays is the practice of adults indulging in self-poisoning which, when successful, is **suicide**, or when unsuccessful, is either attempted suicide, or **parasuicide**, when only a gesture is performed (see **16.2**).

1.0 Introduction

Notes

1.0 Introduction

Notes

1.0 Introduction

Notes

2.0 Epidemiology

2.0 Epidemiology

In Britain, as in most other European countries, North America and Australia, poisoning as a medical problem is predominantly acute.

2.1 Hospital admissions and deaths—England and Wales (Fig.1)

Taking England and Wales as an example, what has taken place over the last two or three decades has been described as an 'epidemic' of self-poisoning. During 1956, hospital admissions for acute poisoning numbered about 20 000, whereas by 1978 this

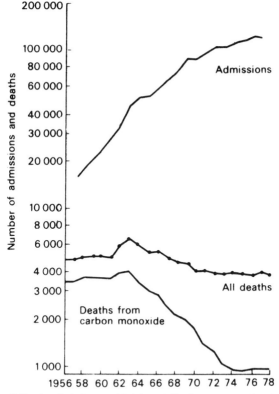

Fig. 1 *Yearly admissions and total mortality from acute poisoning in England and Wales 1956-78.*

figure had risen progressively to over 120 000. Interestingly enough, the total mortality from poisoning remained almost constant throughout this period (Fig. 1). Further sub-division of these figures has disclosed that children under 5 years of age accounted for about 20 000 of these hospital admissions each year, but reassuringly, this total has recently tended to level out (Fig. 2). Despite the classification of the official statistical returns, which suggest that a large proportion of the adult cases are accidental, closer probing of the circumstances points to there being a purposeful intent in many of them. At the same time it is accepted that homicide by poisoning is nowadays rare in Britain, possibly because most murderers are impulsive and poisoning usually demands some advance planning. Detection and apprehension of the culprit is the rule, rather than the exception.

Many of those people who kill themselves by poisoning are found dead before they can be taken to hospital. Presumably they are so determined to die that they make sure not to be thwarted in the process. As the hospital mortality figures have remained almost constant whilst the admissions have risen (Fig. 1), it may be deduced that the majority of these self-inflicted casualties are not truly suicidally inclined; most of them are so mildly affected that they leave hospital by the next day, or the day after.

2.2. Statistics elsewhere

The epidemiological statistics for England and Wales are reflected elsewhere; Scotland is similar, *pro rata* with its population, and this deplorable social pattern is reproduced, so far as one can judge by the statistics, in almost every one of the other so-called 'developed' countries.

Reliable statistics are not so readily collated from what is termed the Third World, but observation points to self-poisoning being far less conspicuous. Maybe, when the forces of nature render survival against inevitable adversity much less likely, so there is less incentive to engage in these self-immolating postures.

2.3 Child poisoning

In the 'developed' countries, small children have become increasingly protected against the depredations of malnutrition, infection and trauma. Proportionately, then, the risks which youngsters

2.0 Epidemiology

2.3 Child poisoning

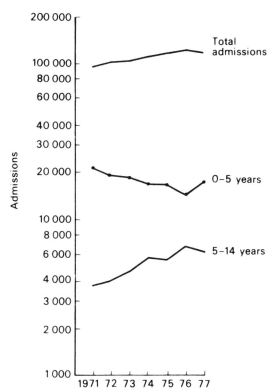

Fig. 2 *Admissions from hospital for acute poisoning in children in England and Wales 1971-77.*

attract by their careless ingestion of toxic substances become more conspicuous.

In England and Wales about 130 children under the age of 10 die each year from poisoning, with carbon monoxide to blame for no less than 100 of these. It must nevertheless be pointed out that this latter certification includes many fatalities not primarily from the gas, but being deaths from carboxyhaemoglobinaemia brought about secondarily by fires, explosions, etc.

Viewed against the hospital admission figures for these young-sters (some 20 000 per year), the level of mortality is remarkably low. What is more, when it is discovered that most of them stay in hospital just overnight, it must be concluded that few of them are really ill from poisons and, indeed, that many of them are taken into the wards with no more than suspected poisoning and just as an understandable precaution.

In the Third World, as could be expected, the extent of child poisoning is not at all well documented, but experience would indicate that, in relation to disease and death from other causes, poisoning among youngsters is comparatively meagre in incidence.

2.4 Agents involved

It is not surprising that, with small children, the substances which they manage to put into their mouths comprise a multifarious collection of whatever happens to be in the home, or in the vicinity. Even so, carbon monoxide apart, the mortality statistics incriminate chiefly the solid-dose forms (i.e. tablets and capsules) of those medicaments negligently left unguarded and within their reach.

Poisoning accidents to adults, numerically of relatively small extent, can be ascribed to a diverse range of agents, among which toxic gases and vapours feature prominently, along with a few metals, of which lead still occupies a sinister role.

When one turns to the relative immensity of self-poisoning in adults, then with perhaps a little over-simplification the indictment falls upon those drugs which the public believes will render them unconscious; in short, the psychotropic medicaments which are so widely in demand for treating that state of mind — misery, dejection, hopelessness and pain — that conspires anyway to overdose. Some of these drugs, like aspirin, can be purchased freely over the counter. More of them can be procured only against medical prescriptions, of which there would seem to be no dearth. At the present time the barbiturates are not so high on this list since their medical prescribing has been curtailed, but ominously their place has been taken, or overtaken, by the anti-depressants, hypnotics, sedatives, tranquillisers, analgesics and so on that make up the pharmaceutical armamentarium for treating the psychoneurotic states so common in the population today (Fig. 3).

20

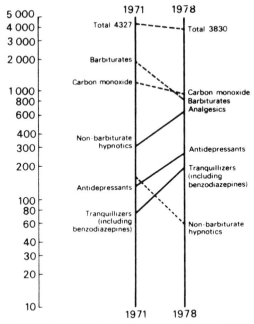

Fig. 3 *Deaths from poisoning in England and Wales 1971-78. Number of deaths where a single agent was involved.*

2.5   Summary

Generalising, then, so far as the developed communities are concerned:

1 The majority of the cases of poisoning for which medical help is sought are of an **acute** nature.

2 In adults, the commonest cause is deliberate self-overdosing with drugs, chiefly of the psychotropic type.

3 Only a few of these patients are so seriously ill as to require active medical treatment, though all of them demand care and attention.

4 With children, the highest mortality is due to carbon monoxide. Otherwise the most deadly agents which they take are medicinal tablets, capsules, etc. The rest of the household products to which they gain access are, in the main, not very hazardous.

2.0 Epidemiology

Notes

2.0 Epidemiology

Notes

2.0 Epidemiology

Notes

3.0 Primary assessment and management: first aid

Contrary to the assumption nurtured by the general public and more so by the newsmongers, the doctor faced with poisoning does not have a battery of specific antidotes at his command and the deployment of these in medical practice is the exception. Non-specific, resuscitative measures are the key to management that is likely to culminate in a favourable outcome.

3.1 Appraisal

Unlike other medical emergencies, acute poisoning is difficult to diagnose from the clinical signs alone. The aetiology is derived largely from the history and circumstances. Someone known to be mentally depressed has been found unconscious with a suicide note alongside and, nearby, is an empty, labelled, tablet container. Or a child is found nibbling something extraordinary that is not normally regarded as consumable. Elsewhere, there has been known to have been an escape of gas at work and a man is brought in coughing, gasping and cyanosed. Accordingly, an accurate if expeditious note should be made at the outset of what the family, neighbours, parents, workmates, police or ambulance personnel have to say.

Sometimes, to begin with, poisoning is not even suspected. Only after resuscitative measures have been instituted does the real cause come to light. Any immediate danger to the patient must be overcome, before time is expended on enquiries, or investigations, to elicit the precise diagnosis. If, however, there is some clue to a condition for which a specific antidote is indicated, this should be earnestly pursued (see Chapter 4, p. 33).

3.2 Assessment

Without being distracted or delayed by the sometimes emotional and incoherent explanations of those who accompany the victim, the doctor's pre-eminent duty is to the patient. Is he or she in imminent danger? If so, the appropriate resuscitative intervention should be launched at once, just as it would be for any other medical emergency (see **3.3**).

In the absence of such a crisis, a prompt yet thorough examination of the patient should be conducted, with particular respect to:

- the level of consciousness
- the respiration
- the circulatory status, including the pulse and blood pressure
- any tremors or convulsions
- the size of the pupils
- the condition of the skin—hot, cold, clammy, pigmented, jaundiced, etc.
- any external marks of injury—circumoral and oral staining, excoriation, corrosion, etc.
- injection marks, if any
- the body temperature taken rectally and advisedly with a low-reading thermometer.

Any other general features should be noted as well, not neglecting trauma, for poisoned patients can be injured by falling, or they may additionally have been assaulted. This assessment should be completed in a matter of minutes and a succinct record made contemporaneously.

3.3   Emergency treatment

This is virtually confined to life-saving measures, thus:

- *Is the patient visibly and spontaneously ventilating to an adequate degree? Are the skin and mucosa of a hue consistent with adequate respiration?*

If so, no aid is needed, aside from putting the patient in a lateral position, with the tongue drawn forward, and seeing that any potential obstructions to the airway are eliminated.

- *Is spontaneous ventilation manifestly inadequate; is there evidence of obstruction to the airways; are the skin and mucosae overtly cyanosed?*

If so, a clear airway should be ensured; any obvious obstructions should be removed, or overcome; an oropharyngeal airway may need to be inserted; ventilatory support should be provided by whatever means are to hand—by the mouth-to-mouth technique (but not if cyanide has been swallowed), by an Ambu bag, or by such other appropriate equipment as can be mobilised.

- *Is the patient unconscious?*

If so, positioning laterally is important, preferably somewhat 'head-down' and with the tongue drawn forward, with care being exercised to prevent injuries from external trauma, falls, hot objects, etc.

- *Is the pulse regular and full and is the blood pressure normo-tensive?*

If not, the foot of the stretcher, or bed, should be elevated by about 20°, to promote venous return to the heart. This, alone, can be salutary in many instances. If not, an intravenous infusion of a plasma expander, e.g. dextran (i.e. colloid, rather than crystalloid) should be set up.

- *Is the patient convulsing?*

Simple tremors are of little concern, but frank convulsions should be suppressed, preferably by an intravenous injection of 5-10 mg diazepam, with dosage according to the response.

- *Is the patient cold?*

If so, he or she should be kept warm, without the over-zealous application of heat from an external source.

- *Has a poisonous gas, or vapour, been inhaled?*

The patient should be removed at once from the polluted atmosphere, with care being taken to avoid the would-be rescuers being overcome as well. Adequate respiration should thereupon be assured, as above.

- *Have the eyes, skin or clothing become contaminated by toxic material?*

If so, the eyes should be thoroughly irrigated, preferably with saline, or otherwise with water, taking deliberate care to keep the eyelids separated; soiled clothing should be removed and wherever the skin has become contaminated, this should be washed, the patient being covered in clean blankets, etc. immediately thereafter.

3.4 Summary

First aid, therefore, is concentrated upon:

- maintenance of respiration
- support to the cardiovascular system
- control of convulsions

3.0 Primary assessment and management: first aid

3.4 Summary

- care and protection of the unconscious patient
- eliminating, as need be, any further exposure

In this process the doctor should not be distracted into taking a detailed history, or collecting specimens for analysis.

3.0 Primary assessment and management: first aid

Notes

3.0 Primary assessment and management: first aid

Notes

4.0 Specific antidotes

At this juncture, thought should be given to the applicability of specific antidotes for, while in practice the opportunities to exhibit these may be few, whenever they are to be employed they should be administered without delay. The types of poisoning amenable to this line of treatment and the corresponding antidotes are given in the following table:

Antidotes available for some poisons

Poison	Antidote(s)	Page reference
Carbon monoxide	Oxygen	85
Opiates, e.g. morphine, heroin (diamorphine), pethidine (meperidine), methadone, dextropropoxyphene, etc.	Naloxone	108
Paracetamol	Methionine or N-Acetylcysteine	91
Cyanides	Dicobalt edetate (or sodium nitrate and sodium thiosulphate intravenously)	169
Methyl alcohol and ethylene glycol	Ethanol	110 and 113
Organophosphate pesticides	Atropine and pralidoxime	121
Arsenic and arsenicals	Dimercaprol	154
Mercury	Dimercaprol	146

4.0 Specific antidotes

Poison	Antidote(s)	Page reference
Thallium	Potassium hexacyanoferrate ('Prussian Blue', 'Berlin Blue')	149
Lead	Sodium-calcium edetate, dimercaprol, penicillamine	143
Iron salts	Desferrioxamine	148

By turning to the pages quoted, details of the relevant poisonings and their specific antidotes, with dosages and methods of administration, will be found.

If the toxic circumstances are otherwise than those given in the table above, proceed at once to **5.0**, p. 39.

4.0 Specific antidotes

Notes

4.0 Specific antidotes

Notes

5.0 General management

5.0 General management

5.1 Respiration

Although the occasions in clinical practice to resort to the specific antidotes just described are seldom, it is vital that, if they are to be deployed at all, they should be brought into action forthwith. That is why they have been accorded priority in this text. More often, though, the effective and only treatment for acute poisoning is that which aims to safeguard the vital functions—respiratory, cardiovascular, nervous, renal, etc. Accordingly this follows the same lines of resuscitation and support that govern the conservative management of all other medical emergencies.

5.1 Respiration

'Dum spiro spero' ('While there is breath there is hope') may be a classical aphorism, but it conveys a cardinal lesson in the care of the poisoned patient, for any deficiency in the oxygenation of the patient, especially so far as the brain is concerned, will put full recovery in jeopardy.

Emergency measures

First-aid for the poisoned patient has already been discussed and, to some extent, reference has been made to respiration under this heading (see **3.3**). If there is no evidence of respiratory obstruction, the spontaneous ventilatory excursions appear adequate and the colour of the skin and mucosae is good and without cyanosis (not forgetting that cyanosis does not present with carbon monoxide, or cyanide, poisoning), then there is no reason to intervene. The patient should be put into a suitable position, usually a lateral one, without any external impediments to breathing, and kept under constant observation, for it is characteristic with poisoning that deterioration in the respiration can come about suddenly, or insidiously.

Where it is apparent that respiration is defective, then the first step is to make sure that the airway is clear. Dentures, or any other objects likely to create an obstruction in the mouth and oropharynx, should be removed and, unless the patient is conscious, the tongue should be drawn forward and an oropharyngeal airway inserted. With someone in coma it is better to introduce a cuffed, endotracheal tube of suitable gauge under laryngeal guidance. If secretions have accumulated in the respiratory tract, these should be sucked out. In addition, if unaided ventilatory efforts are deficient, then mechanical assistance should be brought into action forthwith.

The inhalation of vomit is a secondary hazard. No attempt should be made to induce vomiting in the unconscious patient and, for such a person, the cuffed endotracheal tube affords further protection.

Intensive care

Anyone whose respiration is not functioning properly should be admitted to hospital and poisoned patients so distressed are best accommodated in an intensive care unit. The aim then is not simply to restore oxygenation, but also to provide against the broncho-pulmonary complications that so readily develop, e.g. pulmonary oedema, pneumonia of various aetiologies, collapsed lung, pulmonary embolism, pneumothorax. It has been shown from surveys that the major factor bringing about death in the poisoned patient is respiratory dysfunction.

In the comatose subject, the value of the cuffed endotracheal tube has been emphasised, though care should be taken to prevent the tube from finding its way down the right main bronchus, so setting up a pneumothorax on the one side and a collapsed lung on the other. It is wise to deflate the cuff for an interval of about 10 minutes every two hours thereafter.

The inspired air is best humidified and, where hypothermia exists, it should be warmed as well. On-going bronchial toilet should be entrusted to expert nursing hands.

Complacency should never conspire to neglect of respiratory monitoring. In addition to the routine nursing observations of the respiratory rate and of the colour of the skin and mucosae the use of a Wright's spirometer is recommended. With this device a finding of less than four litres per minute serves as a warning of ventilatory insufficiency. In the presence of an elevated respiratory rate, misleadingly high minute volumes can be recorded and allowance should always be made for this.

More assuredly, measurements of arterial blood gases can be obtained as a guide to respiratory performance, even if the provision of this service repeatedly throughout the 24 hours may

5.0 General management

5.1 Respiration

give rise to logistic objections. The responsibility for the ward management of a patient's respiratory function is a task for an expert, the anaesthetist commonly filling this role, though a physician trained in respiratory medicine may be just as competent. No standard rules of guidance can be propounded, for so much depends upon the individual patient's status. Nevertheless when, in spite of spontaneous ventilation, the minute volume is less than four litres and the levels for the arterial blood gases are unacceptable, then the oxygen intake should be incrementally raised, first to 24 % and then, if there is no improvement within 30 minutes, to 28 %. Thereafter, the inspired oxygen concentration should be progressively advanced with the object of attaining a Pa_{O_2} of 10.7 kPa (80 mmHg), taking care not to exceed an oxygen intake of 50 %.

If, at this point, (i) the arterial oxygen value is still sub-optimal or (ii) the arterial Pa_{CO_2} is above 6.6 kPa (50 mmHg) or (iii) the minute volume is below 4 l min^{-1} (perhaps modifying these criteria where severe lung damage is pre-existing), then mechanical ventilation is essential. Doctors may have little choice over the type of ventilatory equipment which they are called upon to handle, but that which will deliver a variable concentration of oxygen, which will warm and humidify the inspired air, and which can operate on positive, end-expiratory pressures (PEEP) is almost obligatory for use with poisoned patients.

Respiratory complications

Respiratory complications are always a threat to the recovery and survival of patients being treated for poisoning and every effort should be made to obviate them.

Acute pulmonary oedema
This is to be expected when irritant gases and vapours have been inhaled. It can also display itself when drug overdoses have been taken orally, but the extent to which this is due to the toxic properties of the drug, or to over-vigorous treatment with voluminous fluid infusions is not always clear. Diuretics and corticosteroids are disappointing for correcting this type of oedema and more reliance should be placed on ventilation with positive, end-expiratory pressure (PEEP).

Inhalation pneumonia
It is quite alarming how often this form of pneumonia is seen in

5.0 General management

5.1 Respiration

poisoned patients and, in some hospitals, it would seem to be an inevitable concomitant of anyone in coma. No matter what precautions may be devised by hospital staff, the misfortune is that the aspiration may have taken place before the patient ever reaches the accident-and-emergency department.

The chest x-ray appearances are generally indicative of this complication, while the arterial Pa_{O_2} is found to be reduced. The patient may be pyrexial, the more so when lung abscesses are forming, and there may be a lesser or greater element of airflow obstruction.

A broad-spectrum antibiotic is first prescribed for the infection, with metronidazole for lung abscesses, and hydrocortisone, at the rate of 4 mg kg^{-1} body weight, six-hourly for the first 24 hours, 2 mg kg^{-1} body weight six-hourly for the second 24 hours, and then 1 mg kg^{-1} six-hourly for the third day, to combat the bronchospasm. If the bronchospasm is persistent, salbutamol, or aminophylline, may be injected intravenously.

The deficit in Pa_{O_2} may call for supplementary oxygen in the inspired air or, in severe cases, mechanical ventilation.

Hypostatic pneumonia
Basal atelectasis subserving hypostatic pneumonia is frequently encountered in drug poisoning, for to the physical ventilatory inertia of anyone in coma may be added the central respiratory depressant action of the agent involved. Treatment is by active and unremitting physiotherapy to the chest, broad-spectrum antibiotics and, sometimes, bronchoscopic intervention for lobar collapse, conducted by a physician skilled in the manoeuvre.

Pneumothorax
This may be due to clumsy manipulations, e.g. advancing an endotracheal tube down a main bronchus, or an intravenous pressure line intended for the subclavian, or external jugular, vein being misdirected through the pleura. First, any such operative mismanagement should be put right. Then, for reflation, an underwater chest drain should be placed in position and intermittent positive pressure ventilation established.

Pulmonary embolism
Any recumbent patient in hospital, the more so when immobilised as in coma, is a candidate for pulmonary embolism. Vigilance is

therefore a pre-requisite. Prophylaxis is not feasible, though it is wise to keep clear of the femoral artery and, by the same token, the femoral vein, for any arterial puncturing or catheterisation that may be needed. Once embolisation has taken place it should be treated actively, by anticoagulation and, if need be, by surgery.

Adult respiratory distress syndrome

What is more commonly called the 'shock lung' may overtake any severely poisoned patient who has suffered respiratory disablement and for whom energetic respiratory support has had to be furnished. Cardinal signs are tachycardia, a high inspiratory pressure on ventilation, a diminishing Pao_2 in the face of augmented oxygen intake and the picture of pulmonary infiltration on the chest x-ray. This syndrome is life-threatening and of poor prognosis unless discovered early and managed purposefully. Intermittent, positive-pressure ventilation (IVPP) is essential, regulating this carefully lest it should aggravate poor cardiac output. Over-vigorous oxygenation of the lungs should be curbed. Any intravenous fluids should be cautiously infused for fear of overload, whilst the fluid and electrolyte balance should be meticulously adjusted, with both venous pressure and pulmonary arterial pressure lines in position. Any fluid surfeit should be reduced with a diuretic. The place of systemic corticosteroids is controversial unless to relieve bronchospasm, though antibiotics should be prescribed for infection.

Respiratory well-being

Respiratory incapacity can be so inimical to the return to health of the poisoned patient that unwavering attention to the respiratory system must be pre-eminent in the scheme of management. This can be properly organised only in a unit with all the appropriate resources—for respiratory monitoring and blood gas measurements throughout the 24-hours, dependable ventilatory equipment, portable x-ray services, provision for cannulation and intravascular pressure recording, physiotherapy, competent medical staff and, not least, a trained nursing complement able fully to exercise their caring skills for desperately ill patients.

5.2 Cardiovascular system

Another likely consequence of poisoning is cardiovascular collapse, or 'shock', most likely to be seen from overdoses of barbiturates, non-barbiturate hypnotics, opiates and tranquillisers such as chlorpromazine. The antidepressant drugs have a propensity for setting up cardiac dysrhythmias which, in turn, may embarrass the cardiac output.

Observation

Anticipation demands that the pulse rate and arterial blood pressure by sphygmomanometry (or by an indwelling line and transducer) should be noted at frequent and regular intervals, at the same time as continuous record is made of the electrocardiogram. The state of the skin, whether pale, cold, sweating, etc. should be observed and it is helpful to have the skin temperature plotted alongside the body-core temperature. Urinary output, as well as fluid input, should always be charted.

Aetiology

'Shock' in the poisoned patient is nearly always an expression of the disproportion between the capacity of the cardiovascular compartment and the appreciably smaller volume of blood contained within it. Venous return to the heart is thereby diminished and the cardiac output falls in consequence, with peripheral and renal vasoconstriction ensuing, albeit inadequately, in a compensatory manner.

Management

A cold, pale and clammy skin may give warning at once of impending 'shock'. When the systolic blood pressure falls below 90 mmHg, or 80 mmHg in younger patients, remedial action must be taken. First, the lower end of the bed should be raised about 15° to 20°. This simple manoeuvre, by enhancing the venous return to the heart, may in itself bring about the desired response

If not, the circulatory volume should be expanded, by infusing colloids intravenously in preference to crystalloids, or by giving blood if blood loss is responsible. Among the colloids, high molecular weight dextran (Dextran 70) is probably to be preferred bearing in mind that more than one litre of this substance in the blood stream may lower the coagulability. As an alternative, there are the hydroxyethyl starches (Hetaplas) or, better still, a sterile, degraded, gelatin solution (Haemaccel). To guard against overload, these infusions should always be titrated against the central venous pressure.

For 'shock' that still refuses to be corrected by these means, inotropic drugs may then be justified, choosing β-adrenergic and not α-adrenergic agents, for the latter can only influence peripheral vasoconstriction and that has probably come about to the utmost already as a physiological adjustment. Isoprenaline can be given intravenously at the rate of 20 μg min^{-1}; or dobutamine, an exclusive inotrope, at the rate of 2.5-10 μg kg^{-1} body weight min^{-1}; or if there is fear of renal shutdown, then dopamine may be preferred, beginning with a dose of 2 μg kg^{-1}, min^{-1}, and raising this in increments of 5-10 μg kg^{-1} to achieve the desired effect, but not exceeding 50 μg kg^{-1} min^{-1}.

Cardiac dysrhythmias, chiefly associated with overdoses of antidepressant drugs, may disappear once anoxia and acidosis have been dealt with. Definitive, anti-dysrhythmic therapy is called for only when the abnormalities are so severe as to embarrass cardiac output.

5.3   Renal system

There is no sound argument for initiating a fluid diuresis, or for turning to diuretics at all routinely, in the care of the poisoned patient. A few toxins, among which are the heavy metals, may directly damage the kidney and, in this event, haemodialysis or peritoneal dialysis may be imperative.

Nevertheless, for any patient who is poisoned severely enough to be admitted to hospital, a fluid balance chart should be carefully maintained and the electrolyte status should be kept under review. Any deviations from normal should be corrected as soon as possible, not forgetting that renal output may sometimes suffer from a defective functioning of the kidney owing to arterial hypotension.

5.4   Nervous system

Positive efforts to stimulate the comatose patient should always be abjured and nursing care should be directed to protecting him (or her) from any injury that might easily befall, because the evasive reflexes are inoperative.

On the other hand, where the central nervous system is directly stimulated by the toxin and convulsions appear, these should be alleviated by injections of diazepam, 5-10 mg intravenously, or by any other suitable anticonvulsant agent. If status epilepticus is allowed to persist it can be disconcerting and exhausting, even proceeding to a fatal outcome, the more readily so in small children.

Mere tremors can be disregarded, except in so far as they may presage convulsions.

5.5 Temperature

Pyrexia points to infection, for few poisons are themselves pyrogenic. The focus should be located and treatment instituted with a suitable anti-microbial drug. There is little to be gained from routine antibiotic prophylaxis.

Comatose subjects, who may have been left undiscovered for some time without adequate cladding against the climate, should have their temperature taken rectally by a low-reading thermometer. If the finding is unduly low, then gentle rewarming is required, though never from intensive heat sources.

5.6 Summary

In this section detailed attention has been devoted to the non-specific resuscitative management of the poisoned patient designed to restore and maintain the vital functions of the body — without prejudice to the few instances when specific antidotes have a part to play, though never an exclusive one.

For most cases of acute poisoning, successful clinical care is based solely on conservative management designed to protect the vital systems. This supportive regime is equally important, even when specific antidotes are given as well.

Ensuring adequate respiration is critical to the survival of the poisoned patient.

5.6   Summary

- A clear airway should be ensured, respiratory performance should be monitored and observation of the patient should be unremitting.
- Whenever spontaneous ventilation is inadequate, mechanical assistance should be provided for it.
- A constant watch should be kept for respiratory complications and every effort should be made to obviate them.

Cardiovascular collapse, or 'shock', is a common accompaniment of acute poisoning.

- This can often be rectified simply by placing the patient in a 'head down' position.
- Otherwise plasma-expander solutions must be infused intravenously, taking care to avoid fluid overload.
- Rarely is it necessary to resort to inotropic drugs such as isoprenaline, or dopamine intravenously.

Fluid and electrolyte balance must be carefully regulated and renal function safeguarded so far as possible.

Convulsions should be treated with a drug such as diazepam intravenously.

Hypothermia should be gently corrected.

Skilled nursing care, especially of the comatose patient, is indispensable.

5.0 General management

Notes

5.0 General management

Notes

5.0 General management

Notes

6.0 Elimination of the poison

6.0 Elimination of the poison

6.1 Ambient exposure / 6.2 Skin contamination

Logical though it may be to rid the body of any toxin harboured within it, critical observation has shown that the scope for practising this approach is very limited and generally of questionable benefit. Further, the additional physical disturbances thereby introduced may themselves entrain supplementary hazards.

6.1 Ambient exposure

Nevertheless, steps should always be taken to interrupt any continuing exposure, or uptake. Thus, anyone in a polluted atmosphere should be removed to fresh air, without putting the rescuers at risk as well, and if the toxic gas or vapour is exhaled as well as inhaled, then promoting the ventilation may optimise elimination.

6.2 Skin contamination

If a toxic material settles on the skin and/or on the clothing there is a likelihood of dermal reactions and also of percutaneous uptake. Few clothing materials prove to be totally impermeable. Contaminated articles of wear should therefore be taken off the patient at once and the skin should be washed with soap-and-water, or just water.

Similarly, when any offensive chemical finds its way into the eye, liberal and prompt irrigation, with water or saline, is called for. In this process there may be some difficulty about keeping the eyelids apart and there are special devices to facilitate this manoeuvre. Simply putting the patient's head under a running tap does not by any means guarantee irrigation of the cornea, or of the conjunctiva.

6.3 Emptying the stomach

In most cases poisons gain entry to the body via the mouth. Systemic uptake may then be deferred while the material lingers in the stomach, sometimes for hours. In this interval it may be retrieved before it advances too far down the alimentary tract. The classical mode of intervening at this juncture is to carry out gastric aspiration and lavage. The sceptics sometimes opine that more damage can be inflicted upon patients in this way than ever benefit is conferred upon them. The procedure, it must be remembered, is not without its own dangers and, accordingly, it should never be adopted as a routine. Less still should the 'stomach wash-out' be decided upon punitively for the supposed wanton stupidity of the patient who engages in self-poisoning.

6.4   Gastric aspiration and lavage

The positive indications for washing out the stomach are:

- good reasons for believing that a dangerous dose of something toxic has been taken by mouth
- a history of ingestion within the previous 4-6 hours or, with salicylates, antidepressants, antispasmodics and similar drugs, up to 10 hours or so
- absence of vigorous vomiting which, in itself, could already have rid the stomach of its contents

Contraindications always to be taken into account are:

- signs of a corrosive poison having been swallowed, for then the integrity of the oesophagus and stomach wall may have been so imperilled that perforation can easily ensue
- ingestion of paraffin (kerosene), white spirit, petrol, turpentine substitute, etc. For these substances the evils of aspiration pneumonia outweigh their systemic toxicity
- gastric aspiration and lavage should never take precedence over resuscitative efforts

With trained personnel and in hospital, it is possible that emptying the stomach in this way can be worthwhile; in the hands of the tyro and in improvised surroundings it probably does more harm than good.

The procedure to be followed is:

1 In the comatose patient a cuffed, endotracheal tube must be in position beforehand to protect the bronchi and lungs.
2 The patient should be placed on the left side, with the head over the side, or end, of the bed and in the head-down position.
3 The tube selected should be of wide bore (Jacques gauge 30 for an adult); anything less will not afford a free channel for the

passage upwards of particulate matter. It should be lubricated
with glycerin, or vaseline, before use. Care should be taken to
make sure that the tip of the tube is not misdirected into the
larynx. (Listening for breath sounds at the open, proximal end
may be a check on this.) In an adult, a length of about 50 cm,
measured from the teeth, should be consistent with the distal
end being within the stomach.

4 With the aid of a Dakin's syringe, the gastric contents should
first be aspirated as completely as possible. Then about 300 ml
of warm (38°C) water should be run in and aspirated in turn,
followed by further, successive washings, each of 300-600 ml
water, until the returned fluid is 'clear'. In fact this ideal end-
point may never be reached, so when it appears that no more
poison is being withdrawn, the whole procedure should cease.

For the lavage fluid, tap water is satisfactory and saline is
unacceptable. Nevertheless, for certain poisons by mouth, special
recipes have been recommended, namely:

Iron salts
The lavage fluid should contain 2 g desferrioxamine in each litre
of warm water and, finally, 5 g of desferrioxamine dissolved in
50 ml water should be left in the stomach.

Opiates (by mouth)
In each 3½ litres warm water for lavage one potassium perman-
ganate solution tablet (B.P.C.) should be dissolved, but all of this
chemical must be seen to be removed from the stomach before
concluding the aspiration.

Domestic bleach (hypochlorite solutions)
This can be neutralised in some measure by using a 2.5 %
sodium thiosulphate solution for lavage and finally leaving about
100 ml in the stomach.

Oxalic acid
With such a corrosive, gastric lavage is probably better
foresworn, although a 1 % calcium gluconate solution is said
to have a neutralising function.

Cyanide by mouth
In this event the specific antidote, e.g. cobalt edetate, should
always be given first and then, if it is still reasonable to wash out

the stomach, a 25 % sodium thiosulphate solution is advised for this purpose and, finally, it is suggested that 200 ml of a mixture, freshly compounded, of equal parts of a 6 % solution of sodium carbonate and of a 15.8 % solution of ferrous sulphate in 3 % citric acid should be left therein.

Whether it is a practical proposition always to employ any of these refinements to the aspiration-and-lavage procedure is questionable. Of more importance is the manner in which the technique, overall, is executed. No matter how exacting the written instructions may be, the skills demanded on the part of the doctor, or the nurse, can only be mastered fully by precept and example.

6.5 Emesis

Whatever its virtues, gastric aspiration-and-lavage has, in practice, many of the attributes of a barbarous assault, from which, if it is possible, small children should always be spared. That is why, for them, induced emesis is preferred. This appears to be as effective and just as applicable, except when the youngster is unconscious, or is without a cough reflex.

Digital stimulation is probably the simplest trick for bringing about vomiting, but frequently it fails to work and all too often the operator literally gets his fingers bitten.

More dependable is syrup of ipecacuanha, also monographed as ipecacuanha paediatric emetic draught (B.P.C.) and not to be confused with tincture of ipecacuanha, which is a much more concentrated and thereby unsafe solution. Given to a child in a dose of 15-30 ml, followed by a small drink of water, orange juice, etc., the syrup (or draught) nearly always provokes vomiting within about twenty minutes.

If there is no such response, a second dose can be administered, but no more. The success rate is then well over 95 %, including, surprisingly enough, some subjects who have taken an overdose of some anti-emetic agent. So, in the ordinary course of practice, particularly in the first-aid situation, ipecacuanha emesis has displaced gastric aspiration and lavage for children, except when they are in coma.

Among adults the value of ipecacuanha is not so well substantiated, but when proper facilities for washing out the stomach cannot be provided, the induction of emesis by its use may well be attempted.

Sodium chloride and apomorphine as definitive emetics should be totally denounced. They have probably caused more injury and death than ever they have saved lives.

6.6 Oral adsorbents

The belief in the 'universal antidote', a melange of magnesium oxide, tannic acid, and activated charcoal has by now, by common consent, been abandoned, if only because of the potential toxicity of the tannic acid component. There may still be a place, nevertheless, for orally administered adsorbents to counteract poisoning by ingestion. Chief among these is activated charcoal. This is unfortunately black in colour, unpalatable and must be given in unacceptably high doses. Not surprisingly it has little appeal for patients and nursing staff alike. Recently a proprietory preparation of this charcoal in an effervescent formulation has come on the market (Medicoal) and interest in oral adsorbent therapy has thereby been revived.

Dosage, however, still remains an objection. While 10 g of this new preparation may be sufficient to inactivate, say, 40 tablets of imipramine, each of 25 mg, no less than 50-100 g of charcoal would have to be swallowed to deal with an overdose of paracetamol. What is more, if given after ipecacuanha as an emetic, or methionine as an antidote, these substances, too, could be rendered ineffective.

Summarising, then, it would seem that there might be some value in offering this charcoal by mouth as an adsorbent for some ingested poisons, (a) provided that it is not regarded as a substitute for emesis, or for gastric aspiration and lavage; (b) so long as it reaches the stomach within an hour or so of the poison being taken, for after that it soon loses its effect; and (c) whenever the patient is not deterred by being given a mass of this charcoal that is five times the weight of the poison already in the stomach.

6.7 Forced diuresis

Once a toxic agent has become distributed throughout the tissues and organs of the body its deleterious influence will persist until (a) it is neutralised by an antidote; (b) it is metabolically inactivated by the enzyme systems to which it is susceptible; (c) it is voided unchanged in the urine or faeces, or it is exhaled in the breath, etc., or (d) it becomes sequestered harmlessly somewhere in the body, e.g. in the skeleton, adipose tissue, etc. Among these possibilities, antidotes have been referred to in **4.0**, and it is agreed that their scope is limited. So far no practical methods have been designed for artificially augmenting the process of metabolic inactivation or, to more than a very limited extent, that of sequestration. Which leaves the concept of accelerating the excretion of the unchanged toxin still to be considered. By analogy, as it were to percolation, the idea gained currency that, so long as the renal function could be relied upon, the instillation of more fluid into the body would result not only in more urine being passed, but also in the removal of more of the toxin dissolved in it. Man, however, does not conform to this elementary physical model, a state of affairs that became obvious only after, probably, some thousands of poisoned patients had undergone the rigours of this forceful diuresis, without necessarily emerging unscathed.

For the majority of drugs taken in overdose, only a small proportion is excreted via the kidneys in the form of the unchanged molecule. Usually their action is terminated more by metabolic degradation. Diuresis will not, therefore, modify their duration of effect. Moreover, the kidney is not, after all, a simple filter; the renal tubules possess a faculty for reabsorbing some of that material that reaches them after glomerular filtration.

Taking these various factors into account it has been concluded that, therapeutically, forced diuresis may assist the poisoned patient only when salicylates, barbitone, phenobarbitone, quinine and possibly some of the amphetamine-type drugs are present in overdose. In other circumstances it is pointless.

More so, the pH reaction of the urine may alter the degree to which this diuresis encourages drug excretion. The salicylates, barbitone and phenobarbitone may be regarded as weak acids. In an alkaline medium they are ionised to a greater extent. When

6.7 Forced diuresis

this state of affairs obtains in the renal tubules there is less reabsorption, for it is only the unionised molecules, being more lipid-soluble, that pass at all readily through the cell membrane of the tubular epithelium so as to regain the general circulation. In practice, advantage is taken of this characteristic in the technique of forced *alkaline* diuresis.

By contrast, quinine and the amphetamines behave as weak bases. For them, ionisation is enhanced and tubular reabsorption is minimised in an acid medium. So for overdoses of these drugs, forced *acid* diuresis may be advantageous.

Indications and contraindications
There is no justification at all in turning to diuresis as a treatment for overdose from any drugs except those expressly listed above.

Before engaging in diuresis:

- the diagnosis must be certain. Analytically the presence of the supposed drug must be confirmed and its plasma concentration measured. This latter should be in excess of 100 mg litre for either of the two barbiturates, or above 500 mg litre for salicylates. For the few remaining drugs, no critical levels have been postulated
- the kidneys must be functioning normally and this must be ascertained beforehand
- shock, or cardiac failure, must not be present
- pulmonary oedema must be absent

Procedure
The above rules having been observed, then:

1 A urethral catheter should be in place and the fluid balance should be assiduously charted. At frequent intervals, the urinary pH should be noted.
2 A central venous pressure line should be set up with provision, on the chart, for its readings to be successively recorded.
3 Before the diuresis is started, the electrolyte, urea, sugar and pH levels of the blood should be measured and any anomalies corrected, so far as is possible. The arterial blood gases should also be checked.
4 The foregoing all having been completed, the intravenous infusion can then be commenced, with 500 ml of 5 % dextrose, 500 ml of 1.2 % or 1.4 % sodium bicarbonate and 500 ml of

6.7 Forced diuresis

5 % dextrose again, all in the first hour (for forced *acid* diuresis, the cycle should be 1 litre of 5 % dextrose, followed by 500 ml of 0.9 % sodium chloride containing 10 g arginine, or lysine, hydrochloride. Or ammonium chloride can sometimes be given orally at the rate of 4 g every 2 hours).

5 To each 500 ml infusion bag, 1 gram (*13.5 mol*) of potassium chloride should be added, the amount thereafter being adjusted according to the plasma potassium levels as repeatedly checked.

6 If, at the conclusion of the above cycle, less than 200 ml of urine have been passed, the infusion should be withheld until renal function has been reassessed, or until it is clear that dehydration is the explanation.

7 Thereafter, the same routine should be followed, the infusion rate being modified so that the urine flow is around 500 ml per hour, though at the start this may be encouraged by the intravenous injection of 20 mg frusemide.

8 The pH of the urine should be tested every 15-30 minutes throughout the course of this procedure and kept within the range of pH 7.5-8.5, by varying the amount of bicarbonate infused. Studies have shown that, in the cause of drug excretion, the alkalinity of the urine is more important than its volume.

9 Likewise the blood should be monitored for its reaction and its electrolytes, at intervals not exceeding two hours, with the prompt correction of any abnormalities. The plasma pH should not be allowed to rise above 7.6.

10 Finally, a watch should be kept for any signs of pulmonary oedema, though, so long as the central venous pressure is kept within normal limits, this is unlikely to arise.

(For *acid* diuresis, which in practice is seldom needed, the urinary pH should be kept between 5.5 and 6.5.)

Precautions

In the light of the detailed stipulations enumerated here for carrying out forced diuresis and the exacting control that must be constantly exercised over its performance, it is obviously a procedure that should never be entered upon lightly. Nor should it be contemplated except where all the resources for intensive care are available. There is no standard scheme which will guarantee both success and freedom from misadventure and, notwithstanding all the respect paid to instrumental and analytical monitoring, the clinical state of the patient must be kept constantly under surveillance, for this, ultimately, is the arbiter by which to continue, to modify, or to discontinue the manoeuvre.

6.8   Dialysis

Bearing in mind the limitations and foibles of diuresis it is understandable that toxicologists should turn to dialysis which, in principle at least, should enable toxins to be more dramatically extracted from the body. Over the years, moreover, the medical literature has been replete with success stories in which haemodialysis is claimed to have saved the lives of profoundly poisoned patients. Too often, though, these accounts have been no more than descriptive and without quantitative substantiation. Controlled clinical trials, moreover, have been impracticable. Laboratory experiments have shown that most of the drugs taken in overdose do not pass readily from the plasma and through the dialysis membranes in current use. Protein binding interferes to some extent. Moreover, even when total clearance of the cardiovascular compartment is achieved, the amount of drug so removed may represent only a fraction of the total body load.

For haemodialysis to be favourably regarded in the treatment of overdose:

- the toxin should be shown readily to pass through the material composing the dialysis membrane
- the total amount of the toxin circulating in the plasma should represent a substantial proportion of the total body load
- the intensity of the poisoning should be a direct function of the concentration of the toxin in the plasma
- dialysis should be associated with augmented elimination by other mechanisms

So it has become clear that haemodialysis is far from being a panacea for treating poisoned patients. It must be adopted only with due regard to the pharmacokinetic and pharmacodynamic properties of the toxin. By such criteria, the principal applications of haemodialysis are:

- severe poisoning with methanol, or ethanol
- similar poisoning due to lithium

6.0 Elimination of the poison

6.8 Dialysis / 6.9 Haemoperfusion

- dangerous poisoning with phenobarbitone, barbitone or salicylates, when forced alkaline diuresis is impracticable
- above all, when the prognosis for the poisoned patient is rendered worse by renal failure

For dealing with overdosage due to short-acting and medium-acting barbiturates, haemodialysis has little place, if any.

The same strictures attend upon peritoneal dialysis, although this procedure has been found convenient occasionally for lithium and ethylene glycol poisoning.

6.9 Haemoperfusion

The limitations inherent in the techniques to which reference has so far been made for disposing of poisons within the body have led to the development, as an alternative, of haemoperfusion. In essence, this is a system in which blood is led from the patient, commonly by arterial cannulation, into an extra-corporeal circuit and so through a carton, or cylinder, containing an adsorbent material. Through this the blood perfuses, being cleared of its toxin in the process, before it returns to the body via a vein. The principal adsorbents selected have been non-ionic resins and activated charcoal in a granular form. Care must be taken to avoid intravascular emboli, pyrogenic reactions, bleeding problems and alterations to the other components of the blood. Various proprietory devices are on the market designed to minimise these hazards.

Indications
As with haemodialysis, so haemoperfusion cannot be acclaimed as the universal answer to all the problems facing the clinical toxicologist. It must be confined to those cases in which:

- the adsorbent has a demonstrable affinity for the toxin
- at any moment of time, the quantity of toxin in the circulating blood is an appreciable proportion of the total body burden
- there is a correlation between the plasma concentration of the toxin and the intensity of the poisoning

Bearing in mind these provisos, haemoperfusion is *contraindicated* when:

- pharmacokinetically the toxin has a large volume of distribution for, when this obtains, even complete clearance of the blood will make little difference to that greater amount of the substance that remains elsewhere in the tissues to exert its deleterious effects, e.g. as with tricyclic, or tetracyclic, anti-depressant drugs
- the natural metabolic inactivation of the toxin is likely to proceed more rapidly than the time taken to install the haemo-perfusion system and for it to become operative
- the toxic mechanism is specific and rapid, e.g. as with cyanides, paracetamol and organophosphate pesticides.

So, haemoperfusion finds its place in the treatment of poisoned patients when:

- alternative modes of management, viz. non-specific support to the vital systems (as described above) is likely to be unavailing, or specific antidotes cannot be brought into play
- the toxin endangering the patient has a small volume of distri-bution in the body, e.g. *all* barbiturates, trichloroethanol derivatives (chloral hydrate), ethchlorvynol, glutethimide, meprobamate, methaqualone, ethanol, salicylates and theo-phylline
- the drug has been analytically identified in the blood and exists in concentrations above certain critical levels, as shown in the table below:

Biochemical criteria for haemoperfusion

The patient should have plasma drug levels not less than:

Phenobarbitone and barbitone	100 mg l^{-1}
Other barbiturates	50 mg l^{-1}
Glutethimide	40 mg l^{-1}
Methaqualone	40 mg l^{-1}
Salicylates	800 mg l^{-1}
Ethchlorvynol	150 mg l^{-1}
Meprobamate	100 mg l^{-1}
Trichloroethanol derivatives	50 mg l^{-1}
Theophylline	60 mg l^{-1}

Techniques
The conduct of haemoperfusion is no task for the amateur, or the uninitiated. It demands the same degree of medical skill and expertise as does haemodialysis. The resources of an intensive care unit are essential, along with the trained nursing personnel that are on duty in such a unit. There must be ongoing and dependable services to measure the concentrations of drug in the plasma, as well as for repeated electrolyte studies, heparin levels and other haematological parameters (Fig. 1).

1 Under strict aseptic conditions, either an arteriovenous shunt is contrived, or other suitable arterial and venous access to the patient must be fashioned.
2 Thereafter, heparin is injected as a bolus into the arterial line and heparinisation is maintained by further infusions adjusted according to the plasma heparin levels determined at intervals thereafter.
3 The extra-corporeal flow is aided by a mechanical pump in the circuit so that the flow rate is, ideally, kept at 200-300 ml per minute.
4 The haemoperfusion is continued until either the patient is judged clinically to have recovered sufficiently — bearing in mind that relapses have been seen after the perfusion has been with-drawn, or when the plasma levels of the drug have fallen to therapeutic values.

Complications
Some fall in the blood leucocyte and platelet count is inevitable. This is most marked in the first hour and seems not to predispose to any sequelae. Minor alterations in the chemistry of the blood are usually recorded, these rarely being of any consequence. Adventitious bleeding can be disconcerting and even disastrous, so that even minor surgical interventions (e.g. cannulation) must be delicately performed, haemostasis must be meticulous and heparinisation never allowed to become excessive.

6.10   Summary

A whole repertoire of procedures is at the command of the physician for retrieving toxins from the body — from the gut before they have been absorbed, or from the blood after they have been systemically distributed. Sometimes they may be life-saving.

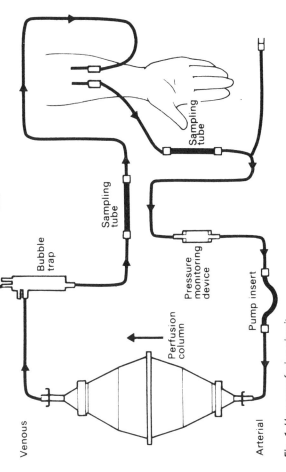

Fig. 1 Haemoperfusion circuit.

6.0   Elimination of the poison

6.10   Summary

Never should they be indiscriminately employed. A favourable
outcome for the poisoned patient depends, so far as the doctor is
concerned, primarily upon the judicious deployment of general,
resuscitative techniques to support the vital systems and, in a few
instances, by the exhibition of specific antidotes. Gastric aspiration and lavage, emesis, diuresis, dialysis and haemoperfusion
are to be called into action only when circumstances justify the
application of these techniques.

6.0 Elimination of the poison

Notes

6.0 Elimination of the poison

Notes

7.0 Laboratory services

The laboratory investigation of poisoning dates back only some century-and-a-half ago, when quantitative chemical analysis first came into being. Its objectives from the start were to resolve forensic uncertainties and, as a result, chemical toxicology was almost entirely medicolegally orientated until quite recently. The transition from the careful, exacting, time-consuming approach, as befitted enquiries into the cause of death, to the urgent demands of the physician, faced with a clinical emergency, was not easily accomplished. Further, the correlation between laboratory findings and clinical status has still not advanced very far. It is not surprising, therefore, that even today the toxicological laboratory does not occupy a prime place in the functioning of a poisons treatment unit. With management of the poisoned patient directed in the main at non-specific, supportive treatment, identification and measurement of the toxin can often be dispensed with, apart from academic interest and, possibly, apart from forensic considerations.

7.1 Clinical monitoring

On the other hand, implicit to the proper conduct of resuscitative measures is the meticulous recording of fluid input and output, blood pressure, intravascular pressures, the electrocardiogram, the rate, depth and adequacy of ventilation and, not least, of the body temperature and state of consciousness. These, clearly, constitute a series of clinical measurements that are essential.

7.2 Clinical chemistry

Allied to these clinical parameters in managing any poisoned patient is the biochemical status of the subject, which can be safeguarded only if there is provision, throughout 24-hours, for recording the blood and urine pH, the plasma electrolytes and the blood gases. In addition kits, or apparatus, for special tests on the ward may be invaluable in some instances, e.g. plasma levels of paracetamol and salicylates, the presence of paraquat in the urine and iron in the stomach contents.

7.3 Chemical toxicology

At the accident-and-emergency stage, for the reasons already advanced, precise chemical identification of the poison is not a

7.3 Chemical toxicology

critical need. Specimens of vomitus, faeces, heparinised blood and urine should nevertheless always be collected, properly labelled as regards the name of the patient, together with the date and time of collection, and put aside, if only for retrospective elucidation, or because of unforeseeable medicolegal enquiries later. These specimens should never hastily be disposed of in the cause of departmental cleanliness and hygiene for, if death should supervene, they may afford, on retrospective analysis, evidence that may then be crucial.

Even in the ward the majority of overdose cases seen are mild enough to be cared for without toxicological delving. Still, there are situations in which toxicological analysis must be undertaken, for example:

- the patient in coma for whom the diagnosis remains in doubt
- on those occasions when the response to conservative management fails to advance as expected
- where active measures to eliminate the poison are contemplated, e.g. forced diuresis, haemoperfusion
- in the certification of brain death, for prolonged coma due to some drugs may be indistinguishable from demise, if reliance is placed solely on intracranial electrical activity as displayed, for example, by the electroencephalogram
- wherever there are grounds for suspecting foul play, whether in adults or children.

The laboratory provision to cater for these demands must be comprehensive, with a range of advanced equipment and skilled personnel, and, if it is to be practically worthwhile, it must also be on-call throughout the 24-hours. Not surprisingly, in few hospitals are the departments of clinical chemistry equal to these demands. Those that just offer a limited repertoire for, say, salicylates, barbiturates and iron, are making no more than a gesture that, however well-intentioned, must be dismissed as being both deficient and even misleading. Logistically, to overcome these shortcomings, it has become the policy in some countries regionally to establish advanced laboratories for chemical toxicology, each serving a number of hospitals*. A system for the rapid conveyance of specimens is then a *sine qua non*, whereas the results can be returned easily by telephone to the requesting hospital.

---

* As this type of service varies from-place-to-place and from-time-to-time it behoves the clinician to keep himself informed of the situation obtaining in his own locality

Screening

At the start the query besetting the physician may well be
whether there is any poison present at all, and if so, what is
its nature.

Some enlightenment may then be obtained by qualitative chemical screening, either of the blood or, more easily of the urine.
Whereas the techniques applied are less the concern of the
physician, the interpretation of the results rests very much with
him. The chemist in the laboratory can only report his findings,
largely in terms of the presence, or absence, of drugs. It remains
for the clinician to reconcile these with the clinical condition of
the patient, to decide between therapeutic dose and overdose
(which is beyond the province of the chemist at this stage) and to
equate the known action of the drug(s) detected with his clinical
appraisal. Moreover the screening programme, however wide-
ranging, can never be absolutely exhaustive, and a negative
answer does not exclude poisons beyond the reach of the screening capabilities. What can be revealing, though, is the discovery
of more than one drug, when perhaps only one was initially
suspected.

Quantitative assays

Ascertainment of mere presence has its limitations. More informative is the determination of the concentrations of the toxic
agents. This puts greater demands upon the laboratory, as
regards its equipment, its analytical competence and the skills of
its scientific staff. Sometimes, too, the procedures may be time-
consuming. Ultimately, moreover, the significance of the figures
disclosed must again be judged in relation to the state of the
patient. Never do figures expressed just as mg l^{-1} give an unquali-
fied answer.

For many of the poisons seen in practice, tables are published
setting out the levels to be expected therapeutically and those
more likely to be consistent with overdose (see Appendix 2).
These should never be accepted as 'gospel', for individual
patients can vary enormously in their reactions. Such tables,
therefore, must be regarded only as guides.

It should also be appreciated that a laboratory finding refers only
to one point in time, i.e. when the specimen was collected. So

long as the patient remains alive, dynamic changes are taking place in the body—by further absorption, by metabolism and by excretion. That is why successive analyses at intervals may be more illuminating about the evolution of the intoxication than one figure in isolation.

A habit to be deplored is casually for the physician to consign a specimen to the laboratory with the artless request 'Poison?'. For chemical toxicology to fulfil its purpose it behoves both parties to work in collaboration, so that:

- the physician consults the analyst beforehand to be advised just what specimens are required and when they should be taken
- when the answers are forthcoming they should not be transmitted disinterestedly on a report form but, rather, they should be conveyed verbally so that their meaning can be discussed.

Drug dependence

Those people who have become dependent on so-called drugs of addiction are notoriously untrustworthy in the histories which they are prepared to divulge to their doctors. In their urge to gain more generous prescriptions they may exaggerate the extent of their indulgence. On the other hand, when they fear that the law may impose itself upon them, they may expediently plead innocence to their waywardness. Quantitative studies on those patients who are dependent on some drug, or another, are rarely feasible. Venepuncture without prior agreement is tantamount to assault and most addicts, at least those who are 'main-lining', so cherish any veins that may still be patent that they will not welcome anyone else venturing a needle into them. That is why one turns to the urine. Not that the collection of such a sample can be left casually to the patient, who may well be ingenious at counterfeiting. A chemically clean vessel must be used and the urine passed into it under direct supervision. Qualitative more than quantitative analyses for a whole range of drugs of addiction can then be performed in the laboratory by relatively simple techniques and it is remarkable how fortifying the findings can be to the physician in his subsequent dialogue with the patient.

Not that these *qualitative* studies on the urine can be transposed in terms of blood levels and they may be criticised in legal proceedings as having restricted validity.

More recently it has been shown that, with the current deviant vogue of glue and vapour 'sniffing', which can put the exponent at risk physically, the diagnosis may be clarified, when otherwise in doubt, by taking blood and examining it analytically for, say, toluene, trichloroethylene and other chemicals for which these people have a predilection. Again, though, the onus is upon the physician to ensure that the blood sample is yielded voluntarily, rather than under duress.

7.4 Summary

- In the ordinary course of treating poisoned patients there is no need routinely to subject blood, urine and other specimens to toxicological analysis
- Nevertheless, it is prudent to collect such specimens, label them and set them aside in the event of possible forensic consequences
- Qualitative chemical screening of the urine may be of assistance where doubt exists diagnostically over a patient who may have been poisoned
- Where definitive procedures are adopted for eliminating a toxin from the body, e.g. forced diuresis, haemoperfusion, then reliable, quantitative toxicological analysis is mandatory.

Guide to toxicological data starts on next page.

7.4 Summary

Interpretation of toxicological data
This guide is based on data derived from the Poisons Unit at Guy's Hospital, London, and from reliable literature sources. Thanks is due to Dr B. Widdof of the Poisons Unit for permission to use these data. The concentrations quoted here are approximate and take no account of factors cited in the text which may modify the individual patient's response. Particular discretion should be exercised when interpreting results in cases of multiple ingestion.

* All concentrations are expressed in terms of mg l^{-1} of plasma except where otherwise stated.
† All concentrations are expressed in terms of μg l^{-1} except where otherwise stated.

Classification	Therapeutic or normal levels —less than*	Levels associated with severe toxicity*
Alcohols		
Ethanol	—	3.00 g l^{-1}
Methanol	—	0.20 g l^{-1}
Analgesics		
Narcotics		
Dextropropoxyphene	0.30	1.00
Codeine	0.10	1.00
Methadone	0.10	1.00
Morphine	0.05	0.30
Pentazocine	0.20	1.00
Pethidine	0.50	2.00
Non-narcotics		
Paracetamol	20.00	200.00 (4 hours post ingestion) 70.00 (12 hours post ingestion)
Salicylate	250.00	500.00
Anticonvulsants		
Carbamazepine	10.00	50.00
Clonazepam	0.05	1.00
Ethosuximide	80.00	—
Phenytoin	20.00	40.00
Primidone	12.00	100.00

7.4 Summary

Sulthiame	12.00	30.00
Sodium valproate	80.00	—
Antidepressants		
Amitriptyline (plus nortriptyline)	0.20	1.00
Clomipramine (plus norclomipramine)	0.50	1.00
Dothiepin (plus nordothiepin)	0.30	1.00
Doxepin (plus nordoxepin)	0.20	1.00
Imipramine (plus desipramine)	0.30	1.00
Mianserin	0.10	0.50
Nortriptyline	0.15	1.00
Protriptyline	0.20	1.00
Trimipramine (plus nortrimipramine)	0.30	1.00
Antihypertensives		
Oxprenolol	0.20	2.00
Propranolol	0.10	2.00
Anti-inflammatories		
Oxyphenbutazone	100.00	200.00
Phenylbutazone	100.00	200.00
Antimalarials		
Chloroquine	0.20	1.00
Quinine/Quinidine	5.00	10.00
Cardioactive		
Digoxin	2.00 μg l^{-1}	4.00 μg l^{-1}
Disopyramide	3.00	8.00
Lignocaine	5.00	8.00
Mexiletine	1.50	3.00
Procainamide	8.00	16.00
Quinidine	5.00	10.00
Hypnotics		
Barbiturates		
Butobarbitone	10.00	80.00
Barbitone	15.00	100.00

7.4 Summary

Phenobarbitone	30.00	100.00
Other barbiturates	5.00	40.00
Non-barbiturates		
Chlormethiazole	2.00	10.00 (oral dose)
Ethchlorvynol	20.00	100.00
Glutethimide	4.00	30.00
Meprobamate	10.00	40.00
Methaqualone	4.00	20.00
Trichlorethanol	10.00	50.00
Stimulants		
Amphetamine	0.10	0.50
Methylamphetamine	0.05	0.30
Fenfluramine	0.20	0.50
Cocaine	0.30	3.00
Tranquillisers		
Benzodiazepines		
Chlordiazepoxide	1.00	5.00
Diazepam	1.00	5.00
Nordiazepam	1.50	5.00
Flunitrazepam	0.05	—
Desalkylflurazepam	0.15	0.50
Lorazepam	0.20	—
Nitrazepam	0.20	2.00
Oxazepam	1.00	5.00
Phenothiazines		
Chloropromazine	0.10	1.00
Thioridazine	1.00	5.00
Miscellaneous		
Bromide	14.00	200.00
Dinitro-orthocresol	5.00	50.00
Ethylene glycol	—	500.00
Haloperidol	0.10	0.50
Orphenadrine	0.20	2.00
Paraquat	—	0.50 (6 hours post ingestion 0.25 (12 hours post ingestion)
Theophylline	20.00	40.00

7.4 Summary

Metal	Sample	Normal levels —less than †	Levels indicating abnormal exposure †
Arsenic	Blood	30.00	50.00
	Serum/plasma	20.00	50.00
	Urine	40.00	200.00
	Hair and nail	1.00	2.00
Cadmium	Blood	10.00	20.00
	Urine	10.00	20.00
Iron	Serum	1.80 mg l^{-1}	5.00 mg l^{-1} (children) 8.00 mg l^{-1} (adults)
Lead	Blood	300.00 (children) 400.00 (adults)	800.00 (children) 1000.00 (adults)
Lithium	Serum	1.30 mmol l^{-1}	2.00 mmol l^{-1}
Mercury	Blood	15.00	40.00
	Urine	20.00	100.00
Thallium	Blood	10.00	50.00
	Urine	20.00	200.00

7.0 Laboratory service

Notes

7.0 Laboratory service

Notes

7.0 Laboratory service

Notes

8.0 Principal types of poisoning

iii

8.0 Principal types of poisoning

8.1 Carbon monoxide

Without in any way discounting the general principles, as previously enunciated, for the management of poisoned patients, a more detailed description is given here of some of the more common types of poisoning seen nowadays, together with a suggested mode of treatment.

8.1 Carbon monoxide

Carbon monoxide remains a serious source of poisoning, especially in the young and in the elderly.

Source

Until recently an almost ubiquitous source of carbon monoxide, certainly in industrial societies, was that literally on-tap in the form of 'town-gas', produced from coal and piped to domestic and industrial premises. Today in many countries this has been largely superseded by 'natural gas' which, by contrast, is almost devoid of this toxic constituent.

Today, the principal source of carbon monoxide is the exhaust gas from internal combustion engines, from which high concentrations can readily accumulate in closed premises. It is formed, too, when heaters, whether burning gas, oil or solid fuel, are improperly installed or are malfunctioning, again notably in closed surroundings, when the ambient oxygen becomes depleted and carbon monoxide is liberated rather than the dioxide.

Most cases of this type of poisoning are accidental, though it is still a chosen method of suicide (natural gas, by contrast, is far less toxic and is dangerous only when it reaches asphyxiant levels) (Fig. 1).

Action

The normally healthy person generates a modicum of carbon monoxide endogenously by metabolism, so that ordinarily the carboxyhaemoglobin level of the blood remains around 1-3 %, being somewhat higher in people who smoke and those living and working in industrial surroundings.

Toxicologically carbon monoxide owes its action to its avidity for combining with haemoglobin at the expense of oxyhaemoglobin.

8.0 Principal types of poisoning

8.1 Carbon monoxide

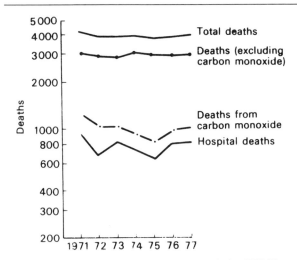

Fig. 1 Deaths from poisoning in England and Wales 1971-77

As the level of carboxyhaemoglobin in the blood increases, the capacity of the circulation to convey oxygen throughout the body is depleted. Tissue hypoxia thus ensues and is intensified by the simultaneous interference with the normal dissociation process of oxyhaemoglobin. The severity of the poisoning is a function of the carbon monoxide concentration of the inspired air and the length of time during which the subject is exposed to this polluted atmosphere.

Signs and symptoms

Carbon monoxide is odourless and its presence toxicologically is betrayed only by the adverse effects it brings about in living creatures. In man, headache and agitation give way to confusion and thence to coma, with hypotonia and hyporeflexia. The early manifestations can easily be mistaken for hysteria. Gastro-intestinally there may be vomiting and faecal incontinence. Some patients complain early on of hearing loss and, more ominously, hyperventilation gives way to pulmonary oedema and respiratory depression. The skin and mucosae may take on a pinkish hue and bullous lesions may appear, particularly at the pressure points. Cardiac irregularities may be associated with myocardial ischaemia and infarction.

86

8.0 Principal types of poisoning

8.1 Carbon monoxide

The old and sick are more liable to suffer from the consequences of carboxyhaemoglobinaemia than those basically healthy.

Delayed effects, which may be in some degree persistent, include mental confusion and dementia, while strokes and myocardial damage may be permanently disabling.

Diagnosis

Although the early signs may not be distinctive, the history and circumstances often point to the diagnosis. Later clinical features are more pathognomonic. Dyspnoea without cyanosis suggests carbon monoxide poisoning. Confirmation may be gained by estimating the carboxyhaemoglobin level of the blood—a simple task for the laboratory—though treatment should never wait upon this investigation.

Treatment

Urgency is paramount. The patient should be removed from any contaminated atmosphere and oxygen should be administered at once, together, if need be, with aided ventilation. Contrary to a belief in some quarters, oxygen containing an admixture of carbon dioxide intended as a respiratory stimulant is to no advantage.

If, in a patient profoundly poisoned by carbon monoxide, prompt recovery is not seen when oxygen is given at normal pressures, transfer to a hyperbaric oxygen installation may be justified. However, it is essential that normobaric oxygen should continue to be administered during transit.

Cerebral oedema may call for an intravenous infusion of 20 % mannitol, 500 ml of this solution being run in over the course of about 15 minutes, followed by a similar volume over the next 4 hours. Alternatively, by way of corticosteroid therapy, dexamethasone may be given, 4 mg three times per day over the first 24 hour period and twice a day over the second 24 hours.

To offset possible cardiac complications, which are more likely in the old and frail, the patient should be kept at complete rest for the first few days, with constant ECG monitoring. Any cardiac disorders should be treated conservatively.

Prognosis

So long as resuscitation with oxygen is organised promptly, complete recovery is the rule, though it is noticeable how often someone who has been appreciably exposed to carbon monoxide may take weeks, or even months, fully to rehabilitate psychologically and to resume the customary habits of life and work.

In older people, persistent brain damage, appearing as hemiplegia, monoplegia, Parkinsonism, cerebellar changes, etc., is frequently seen and may be of late onset, as are mental disturbances that may be as distressing as they are unremitting.

Summary

- Carbon monoxide poisoning is an acute emergency
- Diagnosis depends on the circumstances rather than the laboratory
- Oxygen from the nearest available source must be given at once and ventilation maintained
- Diagnosis may be subsequently confirmed and progress monitored by estimating the carboxyhaemoglobin content of the blood
- Cerebral and cardiac complications are not uncommon and prolonged care and treatment may be required

8.2   Salicylates (e.g. aspirin)

The commonest form of salicylate poisoning is that due to aspirin (acetylsalicylic acid) medicaments containing either this drug alone, or admixed with other agents in a compound formulation. Aspirin tablets are still popular with adults intent upon self-poisoning, but the incidence of child poisoning from this cause has decreased in many countries since the orange-coloured, sweetly-flavoured preparations, devised especially for youngsters, have been withdrawn from the market and since child-resistant packaging has been more widely adopted. Less often, severe salicylate poisoning can come about from methyl salicylate ('Oil of Wintergreen') if this is inadvertently or unwisely taken by mouth, as the fatal dose for an adult is no more than a few millilitres.

8.0 Principal types of poisoning

8.2 Salicylates (e.g. aspirin)

Salicylic acid itself, still sometimes favoured medically as a kerato-lytic, is also highly toxic orally, and is corrosive as well.

Finally, repeated, over-zealous applications of salicylate preparations topically are capable of setting up systemic salicylism.

Actions

Within the body salicylates exercise complex actions on the respiratory centre, on the electrolyte balance, on oxidative metabolism by uncoupling oxidative phosphorylation, and by stimulating specialised brain centres. The narcotic effect, by contrast, is usually minor. The underlying, biochemical mechanism remains far from well elucidated.

Signs and symptoms

With therapeutic overdose, or *chronic* poisoning, the toxic changes from salicylates tend to emerge slowly. With an *acute* overdose, the symptoms and signs may be expected to appear within less than an hour following ingestion. Whilst remaining mentally alert the patient complains of tinnitus, deafness, blurring of vision, ataxia, often with vomiting, and may also display irritability of mood and peripheral tremor.

Hyperventilation then becomes evident, along with hyperpyrexia and excessive sweating. Dehydration may be a sequel, with reduced urinary output. Respiratory alkalosis at the beginning gives way to metabolic acidosis, more rapidly in children than in adults. Semi-coma and even coma may beset younger subjects. In some instances, hypoprothrombinaemia may be detected and pulmonary oedema may develop by transudation through the alveolar capillaries.

Diagnosis

This is usually forthcoming from the history, which can nevertheless be dubious or misleading. Minimal features at the outset can be deceptive, for they can quickly give way to severe illness, small children being particularly prone to this sudden and unexpected deterioration. Confirmation of the diagnosis and careful observation are therefore the watchwords. Qualitative testing of the urine by 'Trinder's reagent' will give a purple colouration if positive. Better still and as an indispensable guide to treatment, the plasma salicylate level should be measured. If the figure is below 500 mg l^{-1}, severe poisoning is unlikely. Concentrations of 500-750 mg l^{-1} suggest moderate intoxication, and above 750 mg l^{-1} the condition is serious.

A low level initially should never conspire to complacency. A repeat estimation an hour or two later can be most revealing, for absorption may be delayed and the plasma level may thus continue to rise. It is also suggested that results obtained more than about 12 hours after ingestion can be falsely reassuring, because by that time much of the drug may have left the bloodstream and found its way into the tissues, more so in the presence of acidosis.

It is also essential to establish the plasma electrolyte profile at this stage.

Treatment

Once the diagnosis is clear it is imperative that any fluid imbalance, or acid-base and electrolyte abnormalities should be corrected.

An attempt should then be made actively to empty the stomach, unless spontaneous vomiting has already been profuse, or more than 12-15 hours have elapsed since swallowing. Children should undergo induced emesis, and adults should be given gastric aspiration and lavage. Gastric adsorbents have to be taken in massive amounts if they are to do any good at all.

So long as the clinical signs are not impressive and the plasma salicylate level is below 500 mg l^{-1}, it may be sufficient just to maintain the fluid and electrolyte status of the patient, orally or parenterally. More arresting clinical signs and a plasma level above 500 mg l^{-1} are indications for active elimination to be instituted forthwith, advisedly by forced, alkaline diuresis (see **6.7**) taking particular care to avoid hypokalaemia.

In those cases in which the clinical presentation is more dramatic and in which the plasma salicylate level exceeds about 900 mg l^{-1}, then it is wise to turn directly to haemoperfusion or haemodialysis (**6.9** and **6.8**).

A watch should be kept on the lungs in anticipation of pulmonary oedema, for which the fluid load on the body should be minimised. The osmotic pressure of the blood should also be raised by colloid infusions and, in the last resort, assisted ventilation with positive, end-expiratory pressure (PEEP) should be provided.

If hypoprothrombinaemia arises, vitamin K1 should be injected intravenously.

In the unlikely event of renal failure supervening, haemodialysis is obligatory.

8.3 Paracetamol (acetominophen)

In many countries nowadays paracetamol is sold in greater quantities than aspirin as a mild, non-prescription analgesic. The public at large is not, needless to say, 'au fait' with the pharmacological and toxicological differences between the two compounds. So whereas accidental poisoning of children by paracetamol is exceptional, it is understandable that adults who might choose aspirin as a self-administered poison are just as likely now to take paracetamol instead. The toxic consequences, however, are quite different. In large single overdoses of over 15-20 g (i.e. about 30-40 of the normal 500 mg tablets), paracetamol can be catastrophic, bringing about acute hepatic necrosis.

Action

Therapeutic doses of paracetamol are disposed of by the body principally in two ways; renal excretion of the unchanged drug, which accounts for only a small proportion of the total, and elimination of the major portion by the same route in the form of inactive metabolites, mainly glucuronide and sulphate conjugates, to which conversion has taken place in the liver. A modicum of the original dose, however, seems to be changed by the hepatic, mixed-function, oxidase enzyme systems into a highly reactive metabolite. Normally this is in such small quantity that it can be readily neutralised by the glutathione already present.

With paracetamol in overdose, any augmented excretion of the unchanged drug and of its glucuronide and sulphate metabolites is nevertheless limited and consequently more of the reactive metabolite is formed, to a degree that is beyond the neutralising capacity of the available liver glutathione. The surfeit of the free metabolite therefore binds covalently to the liver proteins, bringing about acute, hepatic necrosis.

A similar, biochemical mechanism may operate with the mixed-function oxidase enzymes of the kidney to cause renal failure, but in paracetamol overdosage, kidney damage is more likely to be secondary to hepatic failure, as part of the acute hepatorenal syndrome.

These toxic phenomena are not to be found when paracetamol is taken in therapeutic doses.

Signs and symptoms

Someone perversely taking an acute overdose of paracetamol may be disappointed at not experiencing any striking symptoms for the first day or so, aside maybe from a little nausea and vomiting. But, after that, the picture that presents is one of acute liver failure. At an early stage, the onset of such changes can be disclosed by empirical function tests — prolonged prothrombin time, with raised bilirubin and serum aminotransferase levels. Meanwhile the patient may be aware of malaise and abdominal pain, with tenderness subcostally on the right. The disease soon progresses to frank jaundice, with hypoglycaemia and even with encephalopathy. Depending on the dose, spontaneous recovery may ensue, or the hepatocellular necrosis may progress relentlessly, along with disseminated intravascular coagulopathy, cardiac dysrhythmias and renal failure, culminating in a fatal outcome.

Histologically the liver cell damage is at first centrilobular and then may become confluent. Recovery is accompanied by complete restoration of the normal hepatic architecture.

Diagnosis

Clinically the dilemma is to decide whether, in fact, the patient has ingested sufficient paracetamol to warrant being given the antidote.

8.0 Principal types of poisoning

8.3 Paracetamol (acetominophen)

The history, if it can be vouched for or verified, is of great assistance with paracetamol poisoning, for if less than about 15 g (i.e. 30 of the normal 500 g tablets) have been swallowed then there is usually little to worry about. Above that quantity, liver damage is almost certain and with a dose in excess of about 25 g (50 tablets), death is well-nigh inevitable, unless the specific antidote is given in time.

More dependable than the history is a measurement of the plasma concentration of the drug, either by a hospital laboratory running a night-and-day service, or at the bedside by the aid of a portable kit giving a colorimetric reading. To be useful this measurement needs to be ready within an hour or so, for the decision whether or not to give the antidote has to be made urgently. If the level at 4 hours is above 200 mg l^{-1}, or at 12 hours is in excess of 70 mg l^{-1}, or it is correspondingly elevated in-between, the prognosis is poor and will, in all probability, be ameliorated only with the aid of an antidote (See Fig. 2).

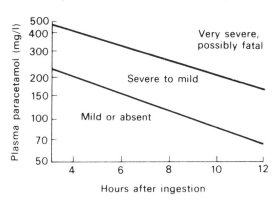

Fig. 2 Measurement of the plasma paracetamol levels gives an indication of the likely prognosis in a given case of paracetamol poisoning and the consequent need for the administration of either oral methionine or intravenous acetylcysteine.

The other tests are those of liver function and they are not specific.

Treatment

Armed with a convincing history it might be prudent anyway to countenance no delay but immediately to administer methionine orally. Even when this might be superfluous it will probably do little harm. The sooner that any specific antidote is given the better the chances of it being efficacious.

The antidote can, in fact, be given in one of two forms: methionine by mouth, or N-acetyl-cysteine by injection. For the former, the dose is 2.5 g orally at the outset, with three further such doses at 4-hourly intervals. If this approach should be compromised owing to vomiting, then an anti-emetic drug by injection may obviate this, or the methionine can be crushed and introduced down a nasogastric tube as a suspension, which procedure should be obligatory anyway in a comatose patient.

The alternative is Parvolex (Duncan, Flockhart) which is a sterile, 20 % N-acetyl cysteine solution designated for intravenous use. The same agent is formulated as Airbron (Duncan, Flockhart) and as Mucomyst (McNeil) to serve as a mucolytic and, when Parvolex is not at the physician's disposal, either of these other preparations may be improvised, for even if they are not necessarily pyrogen-free they are, at least, sterile.

The dosing schedule for N-acetyl cysteine is somewhat complicated. Over the first 15 minutes it is given as an intravenous infusion at a dose of 150 mg kg^{-1} body weight dissolved in 200 ml of 5 % dextrose. Over the following 4 hours a further infusion of 500 ml of 5 % dextrose is run in, containing an amount of N-acetyl cysteine calculated according to 50 mg kg^{-1} body weight and, finally, over the last 16 hours the quantity infused is arrived at on the basis of 100 mg kg^{-1} body weight in one litre of 5 % dextrose.

In the United States it is usual to administer the N-acetyl cysteine orally, the 20 % formulations being diluted to 5 % in a soft drink, the first dose being equivalent to 140 mg kg^{-1}, succeeded by no less than a further 17 doses, each of 70 mg kg^{-1}, every 4 hours.

The side-effects from either of these antidotes are minimal, certainly if given within 10 hours of the paracetamol overdose. After that they are not only ineffectual but, it is averred, they may even aggravate the liver damage.

Ancillary measures include gastric aspiration and lavage within the first 6 hours (before any antidote is proffered orally!), vitamin K 10 mg intravenously daily for 3 days if the prothrombin time is elevated, and adjustments to the fluid and electrolyte status to correct any abnormality of this kind.

Once the liver failure has proclaimed itself, specific antidotes are pointless and intensive care is mandatory.

Neither forced diuresis, nor haemodialysis (except for overt renal failure) can be recommended in treatment, nor do oral adsorbents have any place. A report has nevertheless been published which shows that patients with paracetamol overdose, whose plasma levels of the drug were prognostically sinister and yet who were seen too late to be given an antidote, have fared much more favourably on haemoperfusion.

Summary

- Acute paracetamol poisoning constitutes a medical emergency, notwithstanding the lack of impressive symptoms at an early stage
- If there is good reason to believe that more than 15 g (30 tablets each of 500 mg) have been taken, the antidote should be given immediately
- Otherwise the indications for antidote therapy are based on the plasma concentrations of paracetamol, for the prompt estimation of which means must be immediately available
- Beyond about 10 hours from the time of ingestion the antidote is likely to be not only inefficacious but actually harmful. Late haemoperfusion may then, possibly, avail

8.4 Phenacetin

Whereas at one time phenacetin was a constituent of numerous brands of mild analgesic preparations on unrestricted sale to the public, today it has been virtually consigned to the limbo. Its obloquoy therapeutically was due to its renal toxicity seen when it was taken excessively over long periods of time.

Theoretically, as it is converted to paracetamol in the body, it might, by analogy, be acutely hepatotoxic. In fact this seems not to be so.

Acute overdose of phenacetin, *per se*, is today almost unknown.

Treatment is symptomatic, but the methaemoglobinaemia which appears can be reversed by injecting intravenously 25 ml of 1 % solution of methylene blue, or 1 g of ascorbic acid.

8.5   Phenylbutazone, etc.

Numbered among the non-steroidal, anti-inflammatory agents are, besides phenylbutazone, such drugs as indomethacin, ibuprofen, fenoprofen, fenclofenac, flurbiprofen, to name only a few. They are not the favoured instruments for self-poisoning but, from-time-to-time, patients do take overdoses.

Signs and symptoms

Nausea, vomiting, abdominal pain, diarrhoea, and haematemesis have been described, together with hyperventilation, coma and convulsions, along with renal and hepatic failure.

Diagnosis

This is founded largely on the history, for rapid analytical methods for blood and urine are not universally to hand.

Treatment

Treatment can only be symptomatic and conservative, with emptying the stomach in the first 6-8 hours. Active elimination has nothing to offer, so diuresis should be abjured.

8.6   Barbiturates

The incidence of acute overdose from any of the barbiturates is today much less than hitherto, solely for the reason that they are now not so lavishly prescribed.

Clinically, what are termed the short-acting and medium-acting members of this group of drugs tend to be more toxic than the long-acting ones.

Action

The mode of action of the barbiturates at the level of cellular biochemistry is still not clarified. Towards living tissues they are

8.6 Barbiturates

almost universally narcotic, but their depressant activity is much more conspicuous upon the central nervous system than upon other organs and, within that central nervous system, it is the higher centres that are most obtunded.

Signs and symptoms

With an overdose of any barbiturate there is progressive loss of consciousness and conspicuous depression of respiration. Cardiovascular collapse may be seen along with consequential renal failure. Notably if the patient has been left in coma for some time before being found, there may be dehdyration and hypothermia.

On examination there is coma to a lesser or greater degree, general muscular flaccidity and depressed tendon reflexes. Bowel sounds may be faint, poor, or absent. The pupils are not much affected, except pre-terminally, when they may be fixed and dilated.

Bronchopulmonary complications are very common, tending to be aggravated if coma is prolonged.

Skin bullae may also be seen.

Diagnosis

The picture of barbiturate overdose is indistinguishable clinically from many other causes of drowsiness and coma. As ever, the history can be sparse or frankly confusing. The diagnosis can be put beyond doubt only by blood plasma analysis.

Treatment

Experience in hospitals all over the world has shown that the most gratifying results from the management of patients with acute, barbiturate overdose have been achieved by carefully adhering to the strict principles of conservative treatment (see **5.0**), and by eschewing all stimulants and alleged antidotes. Most of the patients looked after in this manner will recover, provided they are protected against irreversible brain damage that so easily attends upon anoxia.

Emptying of the stomach can yield good returns within 6-8 hours of ingestion.

Forced alkaline diuresis is appropriate only for barbitone and phenobarbitone poisoning, and then only when the presence and concentration of the drug in the blood has been confirmed (see **7.3**). For the remainder of the barbiturates, their metabolic breakdown in preference to their excretion unchanged in the urine renders diuresis pointless. In very severe cases, however, haemoperfusion (**6.9**) may be life-saving.

Summary

- The key to successful treatment of acute barbiturate overdose is intensive, supportive management to preserve the function of the vital centres
- Only for overdoses of barbitone and phenobarbitone is forced alkaline diuresis indicated
- Otherwise, severe cases may well respond to haemoperfusion

8.7 Non-barbiturate hypnotics

The management of patients with overdoses of non-barbiturate hypnotics should follow the same lines as for the short- and medium-acting barbiturates (see above), turning to haemoperfusion again for severe cases due to meprobamate, ethchlorvynol, glutethimide, methaqualone and the trichloroethanol analogues, such as chloral hydrate, dichloralphenazone and triclofos.

There is no merit at all in employing forced diuresis with the idea of accelerating the removal of any of these drugs from the body.

8.8 Anticonvulsant drugs

Like phenobarbitone, the other anticonvulsant drugs, despite their chemical diversity, all have a propensity for depressing the central nervous system, e.g. primidone, the hydantoins, ethosuximide and methosuximide, sodium valproate, etc. Treatment of overdose is essentially supportive, with emptying of the stomach and, thereafter, haemoperfusion for severe cases of phenytoin poisoning and possibly of primidone too.

With carbamazepine, the convulsions that appear may have to be relieved with injections of diazepam, 5-10 mg intravenously, while the vertigo, ataxia, overbreathing, hyper-reflexia and catatonia of sulthiame call for symptomatic measures. Further, the predisposition to crystalluria and renal obstruction that characterises overdoses of this latter drug can be mitigated by keeping the urine alkaline.

8.9 Tranquillisers

Drugs in this category tend to fall into two main sub-groups; the minor tranquillisers, intended mainly to relieve psychoneurotic maladies and the *major* tranquillisers, upon which reliance is largely placed for the treatment of psychoses.

Minor tranquillisers

These occupy many pages of the pharmacopoeias and drug formularies at the present time; the benzodiazepines, including chlordiazepoxide, diazepam, nitrazepam, lorazepam, temazepam, etc. being medically prescribed on a large scale. Both as tranquillisers and hypnotics these drugs have gained a reputation for being much safer in overdose than the barbiturates, which they have gone far to supplant. This would seem to be true, for only immense doses of these drugs alone bid danger to the patients. Yet when they are taken in company with other central nervous depressants, not forgetting alcohol, the additive potency can be overwhelming.

Ataxia, loss of consciousness and respiratory depression generally respond to a symptomatic and supportive regime, while the stomach should be emptied if the overdose has been swallowed in the last few hours.

Active eliminative procedures should be foresworn. Analytical tests to aid in diagnosis have been refined for only some of these drugs and, even so, they are in the repertoire of no more than a few laboratories.

Major tranquillisers

Prominent among the major tranquillisers are the phenothiazines, e.g. chlorpromazine, promazine, perphenazine, thioridazine, fluphenazine, trifluoperazine, prochlorperazine, etc. They are inclined to be more powerful in overdose than the minor tranquillisers and are capable of unleashing bizarre derangements of body function. These include extrapyramidal signs, convulsions, vascular hypotension, hypothermia and cardiac irregularities.

Whilst the presence of these drugs in the urine can easily be ascertained by a colour reaction, their quantitative estimation in the blood is unrewarding in reaching a diagnosis, or in assessing severity. Diagnosis is deduced from the history, coupled with the symptom complex.

To the customary supportive measures of treatment, with emphasis on raising a depressed blood pressure, more by way of α-adrenergic agonists (e.g. noradrenaline) than by β-adrenergic inotropes (see **5.2**), it may become imperative to mollify the extrapyramidal aberrations by giving benztropine mesylate, 2 mg by intravenous injection; the convulsions by means of diazepam, 5-10 mg by intravenous injection; and the cardiac dysrhythmias by the use of lignocaine, disopyramide, mexiletine, etc. For overdoses of the butyrophenones (haloperidol, triperidol, benzperidol), management should be the same as that for the phenothiazines.

Forced diuresis, haemodialysis, and haemoperfusion are of no value in promoting the removal of any of these drugs from the body.

Summary

For acute overdoses of anticonvulsant drugs and tranquillisers, only conservative management is called for, coupled with symptomatic, corrective measures as required.

8.10   Antidepressant drugs

Today society finds itself the beneficiary from the generous prescribing, not only of the benzodiazepine drugs, but of a host of antidepressant agents as well. Since many of the recipients of this medication are, perforce, mentally dejected anyway, they are thereby outstanding candidates for self-poisoning. Little wonder, then, that patients with overdoses of antidepressant drugs figure largely among the clinical toxicologist's clientele at the present time, or that many of them die as a result.

Action

The pharmacological properties of the tricyclic and tetracyclic antidepressants are manifold and include interference with the repletion of noradrenaline and/or 5-hydroxytryptamine into the cerebral neurones, a lowering of the activity of the parasympathetic nervous system, a reduction in the re-uptake of noradrenaline into the peripheral nerves and an ill-defined, quinidine-like action directly on the heart.

Mild poisoning is the rule in adults with overdoses of 600-700 mg and severe poisoning in those who have taken 1000 mg or more.

Signs and symptoms

Drowsiness, a dry mouth, dilated pupils, tachycardia and exaggerated tendon reflexes are seen at an early stage and, with large doses, these proceed to muscular twitchings, convulsions, pyramidal and extrapyramidal signs, coma, cardiac dysrhythmias and hypotension, respiratory depression and hypoxia, acidosis, retention of urine and pyrexia. The electrocardiographic changes may take on a peculiar and not necessarily characteristic form. Delayed cardiac arrest may suddenly occur.

Diagnosis

With a story of someone who has been mentally depressed, who has been prescribed antidepressant drugs and whose signs and symptoms are more or less in accord with the description above, the diagnosis may be made with some assurance.

Any further uncertainty can be dispelled by identifying the drug analytically and measuring its concentration in the plasma.

Treatment

Many patients take comparatively small overdoses of antidepressant drugs and survive uneventfully with no more than simple nursing care and compassion. By contrast, large overdoses are accompanied by a high mortality, so treatment must be prompt, energetic and comprehensive.

With delayed emptying of the stomach due to the anticholinergic mechanism of these drugs there is merit in emptying the stomach, by induced emesis, or by gastric aspiration and lavage up to 12 hours, or even for a longer interval, after ingestion. This can be followed by giving activated charcoal by mouth in a dose of 10-20 g, though the efficacy of this is doubtful.

Meanwhile the usual supportive measures should be put into operation, with particular attention to the respiration. Surveys have revealed that neglect of this aspect has been a major contribution to a fatal outcome. So respiration should be monitored and the blood gases checked repeatedly. There should be no hesitation about setting up mechanically-assisted ventilation if that appears desirable, whatever the age of the patient.

Any acidosis must be counteracted by the intravenous infusion of sodium bicarbonate, for this in itself has been known to resolve cardiac irregularities, the more so in children.

Convulsions should be suppressed by injections of diazepam 5-10 mg intravenously, or by the intravenous infusion of chlormethiazole in 0.8 % solution.

When, despite all these manoeuvres and with acidosis and hypoxia corrected, peripheral perfusion nevertheless remains poor and renal output falls, any hypovolaemia should be overcome by the intravenous infusion of colloids, subject to control by intravenous pressure readings, and there may be no alternative but to venture cautiously an inotropic drug, such as dopamine or dobutamine.

A dilemma then arises if the cardiac dysrhythmias are persistent. Too much deference should not be accorded to electronic vagaries alone. So long as the cardiac output is not in jeopardy, the disarray in rhythm requires no intervention, though observation and electrocardiographic recording should be unremitting. Only when the dysrhythmia is judged to be embarrassing the output should there be resort to anti-arrhythmic drugs and then they should be introduced diffidently, for they seem often to intensify the existing cardiotoxicity of the antidepressant agent already in the body. In desperation there may be no alternative but to apply transvenous cardiac pacing.

Debate continues over the value of physostigmine in antidepressant drug poisoning. Being a cholinesterase inhibitor it undoubtedly enhances parasympathetic activity and, moreover, crosses the blood-brain barrier. Even so, analeptically it looks as though it is non-specific and its duration of action is short-lived. Possibly there is something to be said in its favour in a dose of 2-4 mg intravenously over the course of 5 minutes, repeating this at intervals of 45-60 minutes when coma prevails and respiratory function is handicapped for one reason or another.

Active elimination techniques have no place at all.

Summary

- Acute overdosage with antidepressant drugs is nowadays common. Many of the patients are only mildly affected and recover simply with nursing care. A minority, however, are seriously ill and demand intensive care. Death from severe antidepressant poisoning is frequent
- Successful management rests on a conservative regime with intensive support
- There is no place for active elimination measures
- The respiratory system is particularly at risk, acidosis must be corrected and cardiac dysfunction may be difficult to manage

8.11   Cardiac glycosides

Overdose with these drugs is more commonly of a chronic nature and due to indiscreet therapy. Acute overdoses are seen uncommonly.

Action

The toxic reactions to the cardiac glycosides may be regarded as an exaggerated expression of their pharmacological properties. The fatal dose of digoxin is said to be about 15 mg for an adult and about 5 mg for a child.

8.0 Principal types of poisoning

8.11 Cardiac glycosides

Signs and symptoms

Once a toxic level of cardiac glycoside is reached in the body, so
the subject experiences mental confusion, vomiting, diarrhoea
and visual disturbances. Bradycardia is then apparent, with super-
imposed dysrhythmias, giving way to tachyarhythmias, but the
ECG picture becomes even more distorted in the presence of pre-
existing cardiac disease.

Hypokalaemia is often an accompaniment, as well as acidosis.

Diagnosis

The history and clinical signs are usually sufficient to reach a
diagnosis but, for digoxin at least, this can be confirmed by
measuring the plasma level of the drug by radioimmunoassay at
least six hours after ingestion. Quantities over 25 μg ml^{-1} carry a
poor prognosis.

Treatment

Up to about 18-20 hours after acute ingestion has taken place the
stomach should be emptied, preferably by emesis, for gastric
aspiration and lavage is said to precipitate, or aggravate, cardiac
dysrhythmias. Then a dose of activated charcoal, 100 g for an
adult and 25 g for a child, should be given by mouth as an
adsorbent.

For hypokalaemia, potassium should be given intravenously, in
amounts dictated by the plasma levels. If, on the other hand,
hyperkalaemia should arise, this should be reduced by giving a
sodium resonium ion-exchange resin, 15-30 g orally, or by
glucose-insulin infusions.

Embarrassing bradycardia nearly always responds to atropine
intravenously, 300-600 μg intravenously for an adult and
10 μg kg^{-1} body weight for a child.

Ventricular hyperexcitability is best treated by lignocaine intravenously, 50-100 mg over 1-2 minutes and then 1-4 mg min^{-1} by
infusion, modifying this rate in the light of the electrocardiographic tracing and additionally, if possible, by measuring the

blood lignocaine levels. Alternatively, phenytoin can be infused at a rate not above 50 mg min^{-1}, also under electrocardiographic control.

For patients already the subject of cardiac disease and those showing a persistent atrioventricular block demand artificial pace-making transvenously may be required.

In a few specialised centres it may be possible to turn to digoxin-specific, Fab-antibody fragments in the role of a specific antidote.

Summary

- Acute overdose of cardiac glycosides is occasionally seen in children and adults; more often this condition comes about chronically by therapeutic overdosage
- Mental confusion, vomiting, diarrhoea, visual disturbances and cardiac dysrhythmias characterise cardiac glycoside excess
- Wherever digoxin is concerned the diagnosis can be confirmed by measuring blood levels by radioimmunoassay
- For acute overdose, the stomach should be emptied by emesis and activated charcoal should be given orally as an adsorbent
- Hypokalaemia demands potassium intravenously and hyper-kalaemia should respond to sodium resonium ion-exchange resin
- Bradycardia is overcome by atropine and dysrhythmias should be treated with lignocaine or phenytoin

8.12 β-Adrenergic blocking agents (e.g. propranolol; atenolol; oxprenolol, etc.)

Overdose of these drugs in children can arise accidentally; in adults it may be deliberate, or therapeutic.

Action

By their intense blocking action at β-adrenergic nerve endings these drugs, in excess, exert powerful, negative, inotropic and chronotropic effects on the heart.

8.12 β-Adrenergic blocking agents

Signs and symptoms

These may be summed up as bradycardia and hypotension, sometimes with convulsions and, in severe cases, coma. Bronchospasm may intrude upon the respiratory function.

Diagnosis

This rests largely on the history, for laboratory tests are not very helpful in the emergency situation.

Treatment

As there is some suppression of gastric motility the stomach may profitably be emptied even many hours after the swallowing of an overdose.

Then the treatment should be directed to relieving the β-adrenergic blockage and stimulating the cardiovascular system. With an intravenous pressure line *in situ*, isoprenaline should be infused intravenously at the rate of 10-20 μg min^{-1} for adults, or 0.25 μg kg^{-1} body weight/minute for children, manipulating the rate according to the observed response. In extreme bradycardia atropine, in addition, may be called for, 2 mg intravenously for an adult, or 0.03 mg kg^{-1} body weight for a child. Glucagon is said to be warranted in stubborn cases, given as an intravenous infusion at the rate of 1-5 mg hour^{-1}, as also is a single dose of 500 mg cortisone intravenously at the outset.

If the blood pressure fails to rise despite these measures, then prenalterol, a β-adrenergic agonist, should be given in repeated doses of 5-10 mg intravenously.

Ultimately it may be necessary to apply transvenous cardiac pacing. Any bronchospasm can normally be relieved by a bronchodilator drug, e.g. salbutamol by inhalation.

Throughout, the customary supportive procedures should be adopted, with particular regard to:

- monitoring of the blood gases, with every attempt being made to keep these within the normal range
- acidosis and its modification by sodium bicarbonate

- fluid balance, and using, say, frusemide if any overload should accumulate.

Summary

- Overdose from β-adrenergic blocking agents may come about acutely, or therapeutically
- Clinical features include bradycardia, hypotension, convulsions, bronchospasm and coma
- For acute overdose by mouth the stomach should be emptied
- To restore effective cardiac function, isoprenaline should be given intravenously, with atropine for bradycardia
- Bronchospasm can be relieved by salbutamol
- In severe cases, transvenous cardiac pacing may be essential

8.13   Quinine; quinidine

The two compounds differ physically only in their optical isomerism, but in relation to living systems quinidine is reputed to be the more toxic.

Overdose of quinine is not encountered so frequently now that there is less demand for it as an abortifacient. Quinidine overdose is nearly always therapeutic in origin.

Action

Both of these drugs are muscular depressants, skeletally and myocardially, and both are rapidly excreted.

Signs and symptoms

Symptomatically 'cinchonism' is distinctive, with its headache, nausea, ringing in the ears, ataxia, vomiting, diarrhoea and abdominal pain. Vision can be blurred and there may be diplopia, photophobia and actual loss of visual acuity.

Tachycardia is associated with cardiac arrhythmias and a fall of blood pressure and, on the electrocardiogram, a widening of the QRS complex and a flattening of the T-waves are to be seen.

There may be rapid, shallow breathing, collapse and coma.

Certain idiosyncratic individuals may display these symptoms on quite small doses.

Diagnosis

This is nearly always based on the history and, although plasma levels can be measured, the urgency for treatment precludes such investigations except retrospectively.

Treatment

As spontaneous vomiting from quinine and quinidine can be profuse there is little point in actively emptying the stomach. Forced acid diuresis should encourage excretion but, in practice, by the time this procedure can be established, physiological elimination is nearly always already well advanced.

General supportive measures are the mainstay of treatment with the added manoeuvre of bilateral, stellate ganglion blockade by direct injection of a local anaesthetic to offset visual damage, even though the efficacy of this intervention is today being questioned.

Summary

- Quinine and quinidine overdose give rise to headache, tinnitus, ataxia, vomiting and diarrhoea, along with visual disturbances
- The mainstay of treatment is general, supportive measures
- Early injection of the stellate ganglia bilaterally by means of a local anaesthetic may offset visual damage

8.14   Opiate drugs

Under this heading opium, morphine, diamorphine (heroin), pethidine (meperidine), methadone, pentazocine, dextropropoxyphene, dihydrocodeine and pharmacologically related drugs—the so-called 'narcotic analgesics'—are considered together. Besides being potent in the relief of pain they all have a capacity for bringing about drug dependence and, on this account, their manufacture, storage, sale and supply are rigidly regulated by law.

Overdose can arise as a therapeutic excess, from deliberate self-poisoning and, in addicts, from careless self-injection.

Action

Associated with their central, analgesic effect is the property in all of these drugs to depress the central nervous system generally and the respiratory centre in particular. Many of them also stimulate the oculomotor centre.

Signs and symptoms

The triad of coma, profound respiratory depression and pinpoint pupils is diagnostic, often accompanied by cyanosis. The skeletal muscles are usually flaccid, though there may be muscle twitchings and convulsions. Cardiovascular collapse is not so conspicuous, but acute pulmonary oedema may bring about sudden death.

Diagnosis

The circumstances nearly always indicate the diagnosis and, in addicts, the puncture marks of injections lend support to the presumption.

The detection of any of these drugs in the urine affords additional evidence and sometimes it is possible to measure blood levels.

Treatment

This is a matter of urgency and should never be deferred pending the results of analysis. To reverse the coma and respiratory depression, the specific antidote, naloxone, should be given intravenously (or intramuscularly if this is not possible) at once in a dose of 0.4-0.8 mg, or proportionately in children in a dose of 0.005-0.01 mg kg^{-1} body weight. Within minutes there should be an impressive improvement in spontaneous respiration and level of consciousness. The antidote should be repeated if the response is other than salutary. Failure then to improve should suggest some other cause for the patient's condition. As the influence of the antidote wanes after about 4 hours, successive doses may be required to maintain the improvement for as long as the effect of the opiate overdose persists.

Whenever the drug has been swallowed to excess, gastric aspiration and lavage can advisedly be performed up to about 10 hours after ingestion, for the natural emptying of the stomach can be sluggish, but bronchial aspiration is always a risk in this process unless great care is taken to preclude it.

Crucial though naloxone may be in the management of any opiate overdose it does not obviate the need for intensive, supportive therapy as well. If pulmonary oedema supervenes, mechanical ventilation by positive, end-expiratory pressure (PEEP) may be vital.

It should be emphasised that whenever an overdose has been taken of a pharmaceutical formulation in which dextropropoxyphene and paracetamol have been combined (e.g. as in Distalgesic), the opiate excess claims first priority for treatment with naloxone, the antidote for the paracetamol following it.

Summary

- Overdose of morphine, heroin, pethidine, methadone and related drugs is a common misadventure among drug addicts
- Coma and respiratory depression should be reversed by injections of naloxone, repeated as needed. If there is no response to this antidote the diagnosis should be reviewed
- In addition there should be general, supportive care, the risk of acute pulmonary oedema always being borne in mind

8.15   Alcohols

Contrary to popular belief the alcohols are, in general, depressants of the central nervous system and overdose is almost invariably due to over-imbibing.

It should be remembered that 'methylated spirits' are composed very largely of ethanol, with the admixture of only a small percentage of methanol.

8.0 Principal types of poisoning

8.15 Alcohols

Action

With ethanol, the central effects are closely dose-related, proceeding from the higher cerebral areas, to the brain stem and then successively via the spinal nerves to the medullary centres.

Methanol is less depressant than ethanol to the central nervous system, but it has a singular capacity for damaging the eye. Its adverse reactions are attributed to its metabolic transformation to formaldehyde and formic acid in the body.

Signs and symptoms

To begin with, ethanol brings about a change of mood, varying somewhat with the personality, but generally taking the form of light-heartedness, excitement and elation, even aggressiveness, together with ataxia that may be subjectively imperceptible. This can proceed to sensory loss, slow reaction time and overt incoordination. Vision may be blurred, or diplopic. Finally muscular flaccidity, depressed tendon reflexes, stupor, coma and respiratory depression, with attendant circulatory failure are seen.

Acute methanol intoxication is clinically dissimilar. The drowsiness and stupor are postponed for some 12-36 hours, when vomiting, abdominal pain and ataxia first beset the patient and may culminate in coma. Then it is found that visual loss has taken place and that metabolic acidosis has become established.

Diagnosis

The history can be unreliable and disconcerting, though an account of obviously intemperate drinking, more so from others than the subject himself, can explain the patient's predicament.

Breath tests, as used by the police, serve as a primary screen by which to decide initially whether excessive alcohol has been taken, but as yet the findings cannot always be transposed reliably in terms of blood levels. Analysis of the blood for its ethanol content, by gas chromatography for choice, is simple, reliable and reproducible, though the sample should be stored, subsequent to collection, so as to prevent evaporation and to avoid microbiological activity modifying its content.

8.0   Principal types of poisoning

8.15   Alcohols

The blood levels may be correlated with the degree of intoxication as follows:

500-1500 mg l^{-1} mild
1500-3000 mg l^{-1} moderate
3000-5000 mg l^{-1} severe
Over 5000 mg l^{-1} coma and impending death

Even so, these figures must not be accepted too literally, for different people display quite different behaviour from the same levels, possibly owing to their pre-existing drinking habits.

For methanol, a blood level above 500 mg l^{-1}, together with an increased anion gap, betokens a dangerous plight.

Treatment

For *acute ethanol intoxication* the keystone to medical care is intensive supportive therapy, including gastric aspiration and lavage, if copious vomiting has not occurred spontaneously. Bronchial aspiration, especially of vomitus, is always likely, unless careful precautions are taken against it. Hypoglycaemia requires oral, or intravenous, glucose, but glucagon is quite ineffective. In some instances naloxone seems to lighten the coma and fructose, by the part it plays in carbohydrate metabolism, is claimed to be advantageous, in a dose of 200 g given as an intravenous infusion of a 40 % solution over the course of 30 minutes.

In severe cases, haemodialysis, or haemoperfusion, may assist in removing the ethanol from the body.

For *methanol poisoning*, gastric aspiration and lavage should be undertaken within four hours of ingestion. Acidosis should be treated with sodium bicarbonate intravenously. More fundamentally, the metabolism of the methanol to the toxic formaldehyde and formic acid should be arrested so far as possible by administering ethanol to serve as a preferential substitute for the alcohol dehydrogenase. First 50 g of ethanol are given by mouth and then 10-12 g hour^{-1} are infused intravenously, regulating this rate in order to maintain a blood ethanol level between 1000-2000 mg l^{-1} under analytical surveillance.

Wherever it appears that the amount of methanol taken is likely to have exceeded 30 ml, or if the metabolic acidosis is not reversed by sodium bicarbonate, or where there are signs of damage to the vision, haemodialysis should be undertaken.

The promise of 4-methyl pyrazole as an alcohol dehydrogenase competitor, or of folic acid to encourage the conversion of formate to carbon dioxide, has not yet been sufficiently validated for routine clinical application.

8.16   Ethylene glycol

Ethylene glycol may be regarded as a polyhydroxy-alcohol. In itself it appears to be relatively non-toxic, but deaths have come about from its injudicious incorporation into medicaments and, today, it is sold on a large scale as the principal constituent of many commercial antifreeze products for water-cooled, internal combustion engines.

Action

An oral dose of about 100 ml, or more, of ethylene glycol is to be viewed as dangerous, though recovery has taken place from much larger quantities.

In the liver and, to a lesser degree, in the kidneys, ethylene glycol undergoes an elaborate metabolism with the formation of aldehydes, glycolate, oxalate and lactic acid.

Signs and symptoms

To begin with the clinical picture resembles that of ethanol intoxication, which may explain its attraction to undiscriminating imbibers. After a while there is nausea, vomiting, haematemesis, tetanic muscular contractions, depression of the tendon reflexes, convulsions, eye changes and coma.

Unchecked, these reactions give way to tachycardia, tachypnoea, congestive cardiac failure and pulmonary oedema.

At this stage there may be pain and tenderness in the renal area and acute tubular necrosis.

8.0 Principal types of poisoning

8.16 Ethylene glycol

Diagnosis

Apart from the history, gastric aspiration may yield stomach contents bearing the tell-tale, bluish colouration of antifreeze products.

Investigations then show a neutrophil leucocytosis, a low serum level of bicarbonate and calcium, an elevated serum potassium concentration and a dilute urine with proteinuria, microscopic haematuria and calcium oxalate crystalluria.

If a lumbar puncture is performed, the cerebrospinal fluid has the same characteristics as are seen in meningoencephalitis. Given the requisite laboratory facilities the serum levels of ethylene glycol and oxalic acid may be estimated.

Post-mortem examination in fatal cases discloses diffuse cerebral oedema and the deposition in the meninges of calcium oxalate crystals. The heart is dilated, with the features of myocarditis, while the lungs are grossly oedematous and petechiae are widely distributed.

Renal degeneration is tubular more than glomerular and proximal more than distal, with deposits of calcium oxalate crystals.

Treatment

If the patient presents with a few hours of swallowing the ethylene glycol, then gastric aspiration and lavage should be carried out and energetic supportive treatment should be mobilised. Sodium bicarbonate must be given to rectify the acidosis, often in immense doses, though the hypernatraemia thus induced may lead to fluid retention, predisposing to 'shock lung'. Bearing this in mind, mechanical ventilation may have to be introduced early on.

Where the hypernatraemia is unduly elevated it may have to be lowered by haemodialysis, and hypocalcaemia requires calcium gluconate intravenously.

Just as in methanol poisoning, ethanol will compete metabolically with ethylene glycol in the body to limit the liberation of the toxic metabolites. 50 g of ethanol must be given orally immediately

after emptying the stomach, and the administration of this antidote should be continued as an intravenous infusion of about
10-12 g per hour, again regulating this rate to keep the blood level
at 1000-2000 mg l^{-1}.

Once renal damage is apparent, dialysis is obligatory and the
ethanol infusion will have to be raised proportionally. Ethylene
glycol, as well as its metabolites, will be dialysed at the same
time, but not the calcium oxalate. It is said that peritoneal dialysis
is preferable to haemodialysis in this situation.

Summary

- Among the alcohols, ethanol is frequently taken to excess.
  Overdose of methanol (as distinct from methylated spirits) is
  uncommon, but poisoning by ethylene glycol taken by mouth
  is often encountered
- For acute ethanol overdose, management is based on supportive measures, along with (perhaps), naloxone and fructose,
  and haemodialysis in severe cases
- For acute methanol overdose, metabolic acidosis must be
  corrected and ethanol administered as an antidote
- Acute poisoning with ethylene glycol ('antifreeze') by mouth,
  with its convulsions, cardiac disorder and renal damage, also
  calls for reversal of the acidosis by means of sodium bicarbonate and ethanol as a specific antidote

8.17   Miscellaneous drugs

The world today is replete with medicaments in profusion, far in
excess of those that have qualified for mention so far in this text.
Any of these can be implicated in poisoning, whether of children
or of adults. To tailor treatment in each and every instance is
superfluous. They are all likely to respond to the same sort of
management that has been described so far, viz. general supportive care to the vital systems—respiratory, cardiovascular,
nervous, renal and so on—with the correction of any physiological abnormalities affecting any of them, using non-specific
measures, and with attention to symptomatic relief withal.

8.18   Multiple drugs

The accounts of poisoning given in this book have centred on
drugs one-by-one, thereby simplifying the explanations. The
present-day habit, however, is for adults intent on taking an overdose to swallow more than one drug at a time, devouring as it
were a medicinal mélange, very likely topped up with alcohol as
well. The clinical reactions which then arise may be more confusing diagnostically, but they do not necessarily cause the treatment to be modified. First, if there should be, amidst the medley,
one or more compounds for which antidotes are effective, these
should be given priority. For the remainder, however, there
should be no departure from the standard regime of general,
supportive care.

8.19   Summary

Overall, the treatment of any drug overdose, single or multiple,
should always follow the same plan, viz, to administer a specific
antidote, if that should be appropriate, but always to conduct a
regime of supportive management, intended to maintain respiration and preserve cardiovascular and renal function, accompanied
by any other symptomatic measures that may be expedient.

8.0 Principal types of poisoning

Notes

8.0 Principal types of poisoning

Notes

9.0 Pesticides

9.0 Pesticides

9.1 Organophosphate insecticides

There is no simple answer to pesticide poisoning. The legion of
chemical substances exploited to control pests in agriculture,
horticulture, food storage, public health, vector control, etc., is
extensive and diverse. Toxicologically they do not all behave in
the same manner and they range from some that are almost
innocuous to man, e.g. the triazide herbicides, such as simazine,
to others that are lethal in very small amounts, e.g. dimefox in
the organophosphate insecticide series, and the weed-killer paraquat. Consequently there is no single, or universal, scheme for
diagnosis and treatment to cater for every exigency in pesticide
poisoning. Deliberate self-poisoning with these chemicals is nearly
always by the oral route. In the course of handling them, the skin
is the major portal of entry, the lungs being less often involved.
Each case must be approached separately and, where the exposure may have taken place occupationally, a detailed work history
must be noted, for it is easy to confuse a natural illness with
poisoning, just because a pesticide may have been in the vicinity.
Wherever possible the pesticide should be identified. Trade names
can be unenlightening, but it is now the custom for the approved
name of the active ingredient to be displayed on the label.

Nevertheless, when it comes to treatment, the principles of non-
specific support still hold, with a departure from these only in
special instances which will be referred to below.

9.1 Organophosphate insecticides

Control of insects and other pests by organophosphate compounds is today practised on a global scale. Given common sense
in their handling and reasonable precautions, they should offer no
hazard to man. But working conditions are not always satisfactory, ignorance and carelessness may combine, and accidents
tend to happen. What is more, in some countries, the swallowing
of these chemicals is the favourite form of suicide.

Some organophosphates like the dimefox already mentioned, are
highly toxic, while others, such as malathion and bromophos, are
of almost negligible toxicity.

Action

The prototype organophosphate compounds were conceived as
'war gases' and they could inflict permanent damage upon the

9.1 Organophosphate insecticides

central and peripheral nervous systems. Tri-orthocresyl phosphate (TOCP), a lubricant additive, has been confirmed as the cause of irreversible and fatal neurological damage in man, sometimes on an epidemic scale. Today, the organophosphate pesticides that are released for commercial use by national and other authorities must be demonstrably free from this property.

This apart, these pesticides all have the faculty for conjugating with the cholinesterase enzymes in the body, thereby inactivating them, both in the plasma and in the cells. Acetylcholine thereupon accumulates at all the autonomic ganglia, at the post-ganglionic parasympathetic nerve endings and at the skeletal neuromuscular junctions. Therein lies the explanation for the classical clinical picture of organophosphate poisoning.

Signs and symptoms

The onset may be acute when, say, an organophosphate chemical is swallowed, or it may come about insidiously, for example when someone has been working for some time in a contaminated atmosphere or, more often, when workers gradually absorb the material through repeated contact with the skin. At first the symptoms comprise headache, weakness and mental confusion, soon to be surmounted by more pathognomonic reactions such as vomiting, profuse sweating, hyper-salivation, bradycardia and colicky abdominal pains. Muscle twitchings, or fasciculations, may progress to frank convulsions, while dyspnoea is exacerbated by bronchoconstriction and excessive bronchial secretions. Diarrhoea, tenesmus and urinary incontinence are a prelude to collapse, coma and death from respiratory arrest.

Pupillary constriction is the outcome of post-ganglionic parasympathetic over-action in the nerves to the eye. This can be due to direct corneal contact, or secondarily to systemic poisoning. In default of specific treatment full recovery may take some weeks, during which time the cholinesterase enzyme complement has to be physiologically reinstated by synthesis in the liver.

Diagnosis

If treatment is to be expeditious the diagnosis must be reached without hesitation—from the history and the clinical features.

9.0 Pesticides

9.1 Organophosphate insecticides

Laboratory confirmation, albeit retrospectively, can be derived from measuring the level of cholinesterase in the blood, a sample of which should always be collected for this purpose.

Even then, the figures may carry no obvious meaning, for the so-called 'normal' levels vary considerably from one individual to another. Moreover, gross depression of the plasma cholinesterase may reflect no more than inordinate exposure on the part of the subject, though lowering of the erythrocyte enzyme is more reliable as an index of clinical poisoning.

Treatment

Without dallying while laboratory tests are completed, any patient believed, on circumstantial grounds, to be the victim of organo-phosphate poisoning should be kept at complete rest and a clear airway should be ensured. Contaminated skin should be washed and soiled clothing removed. Atropine in a dose of 2 mg should be given right away, by intramuscular or, in extreme cases, intra-venous injection, and repeated in this manner until a full state of 'atropinisation'—with a rapid pulse (up to 100 per minute), dry skin, dilatation of the pupils and remission of symptoms—has not only been attained, but is also being maintained. In severe cases the total amount of atropine required to bring about this state of affairs may reach 1 gram or more during the first day.

Yet this procedure, dramatic though the response may be, is only partial in its reversal of the toxic process, for atropine counteracts only that excess of acetylcholine which exerts its effect at the post-ganglionic, parasympathetic, nerve endings (the 'muscarinic' sites), without interfering with the surfeit of this neurochemical transmittor elsewhere, e.g. at the 'nicotinic' sites, both at the ganglia on the autonomic nervous system and at the skeletal neuromuscular nerve endings. So as to achieve a more thorough restoration of the cholinesterase function throughout the body, an attempt should be made directly to reverse the conjugation that has taken place between this enzyme and the organophosphate molecule. By the aid of a specific enzyme reactivator this may be possible. Such a reactivator is *pralidoxime*, of which 1 gram should be injected intravenously at the outset, with up to two more doses of the same order subsequently. Little is to be gained by persisting with this form of antidotal therapy beyond the first 24-hours, for after that interval the conjugated state cannot be disrupted. As an alternative to pralidoxime, obidoxime may be injected intramuscularly in a dose of 3.0 mg kg^{-1} body weight.

Ancillary to this specific approach should be other, more general measures. The stomach should be emptied when the chemical has been taken by mouth. The airway should be kept clear, if need be by bronchial suction, and support to the respiration should never be neglected. Convulsions should be controlled with intravenous diazepam, this drug appearing to exercise a non-specific beneficial effect as well.

Diagnosis and severity can be gauged by measuring the cholin-esterase levels in the blood, but this should always be deferred pending urgent clinical treatment.

Summary

- Organophosphate poisoning, which usually arises from occupa-tional exposure to pesticides of this type, or from the deliberate swallowing of them, is usually apparent from the history and from the clinical signs of cholinergic excess—vomiting, excess-ive salivation and sweating, abdominal colic, dyspnoea and bronchoconstriction, muscle fasciculations, and 'pin-point' pupils
- Treatment is urgent by means of atropine, given intramuscu-larly, or intravenously, in repeated doses of 2 mg, until full 'atropinisation' is attained. To this should be added prali-doxime, 1 gram intravenously, up to three successive doses
- If the chemical has been swallowed, gastric aspiration and lavage should be effected and, with topical exposure, skin and clothing should be decontaminated
- Absolute rest should be decreed for the patient, with general supportive measures

9.2 Carbamate insecticides

These are being increasingly utilised as commercial pesticides nowadays.

Action

The specific pharmacological action of these carbamates is similar to that of the organophosphate compounds, with the difference, however, that the conjugation with the cholinesterase enzymes is spontaneously reversible.

Signs and symptoms

Clinically carbamate poisoning is indistinguishable from that caused by the organophosphates.

Diagnosis

Reliance must be placed entirely on the history, signs and symptoms, for laboratory tests for the enzymes are unrewarding.

Treatment (see p. 123)

This is the same, too, as for organophosphate poisoning, but cholinesterase reactivators are definitely contraindicated.

Summary

- Both the organophosphate and the carbamate pesticides act in the same way, viz, by inactivating the cholinesterase enzymes in the body
- Carbamates thus lead to a similar 'cholinergic' clinical picture with weakness, vomiting, profuse sweating, hypersalivation, bradycardia, muscle fasciculations, colicky abdominal pains, bronchoconstriction and excessive bronchial secretions
- Treatment relies on the assurance of a clear airway and the maintenance of respiration, with atropine injections as the specific antidote, but for the carbamates the reactivating agents such as pralidoxime and obidoxime are definitely contra-indicated.

9.3 Organochlorine insecticides

These include, among others, dicophane (DDT), aldrin, dieldrin, endrin and lindane. Being substances that are resistant to chemical and biological degradation these chemicals can persist in the environment, so the official policy now in nearly every country of the world is to phase out their use so far as is practicable.

9.0 Pesticides

9.3 Organochlorine insecticides

Action

All of the organochlorine insecticides function as direct stimulants to the central nervous system, though they are not of high acute toxicity to man.

Chronic exposure encourages the storage of these chemicals in the body fat so that sequestration takes place in the adipose tissues.

Signs and symptoms

Stimulation of the central nervous system gives rise to anxiety, excitement, muscle fasciculations and convulsions, with consciousness being retained. Ultimately there may be respiratory exhaustion and failure.

Diagnosis

Blood may be taken for confirmatory analysis later, but the diagnosis depends almost entirely upon history and signs.

Treatment

Exposure is nearly always parenteral, but if any of these compounds has been swallowed, the stomach should be emptied and a saline purge administered. Convulsions should be amenable to diazepam, 5-10 mg by intravenous injection, though in extreme distress, 'curarisation' with mechanical ventilation may have to be brought into play.

The outcome is nearly always favourable and recovery complete.

Summary

- The organochlorine insecticides stimulate the central nervous system, leading to excitement and convulsions
- Treatment relies on control of the convulsions, usually by means of diazepam injections

9.4   Dinitro-compounds

Such chemicals as dinitro-orthocresol (DNOC), dinoseb, etc., are used as 'winter washes' in orchards and as herbicides and plant desiccants in the summer. Occupationally the latter creates the greater likelihood of worker hazard.

Action

Common to all of these dinitro-compounds toxicologically is their biochemical action within the cell, whereby they 'uncouple' oxidative phosphorylation. Thus they engender augmented cellular metabolism throughout the body, thereby setting up a state of overall hypermetabolism without the intermediation of the thyroid gland.

Signs and symptoms

Yellow-staining of the skin and mucosae serves as an alert to over-exposure but, in itself, this should not be accepted as a sign of poisoning, which is demonstrated by extraordinary tiredness, sweating and thirst, with restlessness, tachycardia, pyrexia, hyperpnoea, loss of weight and collapse.

Diagnosis

The history and appearance together may be sufficiently diag-nostic but, if not, blood should be taken for estimating the dinitro-compound levels therein.

Treatment

There is no specific antidote. Complete rest should be ordained, fluid and electrolyte loss should be replenished, oxygen should be supplied and the ventilation should never be allowed to falter. Tepid spraying for hyperpyrexia may be helpful. The chemicals concerned are metabolised fairly rapidly and, so long as the vital processes can be supported meantime, recovery should be complete.

9.5 Pentachlorophenol, etc.

Pentachlorophenol still occupies a place as a valuable timber preservative, and the herbicides bromoxynil and ioxonyl have similar toxicological properties. Occupational exposure, which is of more consequence in hot climates, is chiefly via the skin.

Action

Pentachlorophenol and its associated chemicals share the property with the dinitro-compounds of 'uncoupling' oxidative phosphorylation.

Much controversy surrounds the liability to chronic poisoning from pentachlorophenol, because of the trace of dioxin which finds it way into the final material during the process of manufacture. This question remains largely unresolved, but meanwhile the manufacturing process is being modified so that the residual content of these dioxins is minimal.

Signs and symptoms

Over-exposure to pentachlorophenol and such-like chemicals leads to a hypermetabolic state akin to that seen with the dinitro-compounds, but without the yellow staining of the skin and mucosae.

Chronic exposure to pentachlorophenol may bring about a skin condition called 'chloracne' which is ascribed to the dioxin impurities.

Diagnosis

Chemical tests are not of much assistance clinically, except in so far as the qualitative detection of the compound in the urine can be diagnostically consolidating.

Treatment

This should follow the same lines as for dinitro-poisoning.

Summary

- Poisoning from any of the dinitro-compounds, from penta-chlorophenol and from related compounds, is characterised by a hypermetabolic state, with sweating, pyrexia, hyperpnoea, tachycardia and exhaustion
- For treatment the patient should be kept at complete rest, respiration assured, cooling measures applied and fluid and electrolyte depletion restored

9.6 Chlorates

The chlorates of sodium and potassium still find favour in practice as total herbicides, clearing the ground of all vegetation.

Action

In the dry state these chlorates are strong oxidising agents and create a high risk of fire and explosion, which is their principal danger occupationally. Workers, otherwise, are at no great hazard, but if someone should swallow the chemical, deliberately or accidentally, it can turn out to be highly toxic, a single dose of about 15 g being lethal for an adult and proportionately less for a child.

Signs and symptoms

Following ingestion the immediate reaction is a 'burning' sensation in the mouth and throat, soon to be succeeded by abdominal pain, vomiting, confusion, methaemoglobinaemia and cyanosis. Convulsions may arise and renal damage ensue.

Diagnosis

The clinical picture, coupled with the history, generally supplies the answer.

Treatment

Within a few hours of ingestion, gastric aspiration and lavage is recommended and then a saline purge should be given.

Methaemoglobinaemia may be reversed by the intravenous injection of 5-20 ml of a 1 % methylene blue solution. Fluid intake and, by the same token, the urine output should be encouraged, unless renal damage intervenes, when haemodialysis is indicated.

Summary

- The principal occupational risk from sodium or potassium chlorate is fire and explosion
- If these chemicals are swallowed they cause abdominal pain, vomiting, methaemoglobinaemia and renal damage
- The stomach should be emptied, the methaemoglobinaemia reversed by injections of methylene blue, fluid intake and urine output should be promoted, but if renal failure supervenes, haemodialysis is called for

9.7 Bipyridilium herbicides—paraquat, diquat, etc.

Paraquat, diquat and morfamquat are bipyridilium compounds which are extensively employed as total weed-killers, though they are soon inactivated in the soil.

Action

The mode of action of these compounds on mammalian tissues is still obscure. A single oral dose of 3 g or so of paraquat may be fatal for an adult.

Signs and symptoms

Repeated immersion of the hands in paraquat solutions, whether as the concentrate or as diluted for use, can cause deformities in the beds of the finger-nails. Subsequent regrowth, however, is normal.

In the eyes the commercial concentrate (usually a 20 % solution) is highly irritant.

Apart from these effects there are few risks to people normally handling these herbicides, subject to reasonable hygienic care. Disasters are met with, however, when someone actually swallows these compounds, intentionally or accidentally. Ingestion of the concentrate then leads to inflammation and sometimes corrosion in the mouth and throat, though spontaneous healing usually follows in the course of a few days.

Large doses can provoke abdominal pain and vomiting and, thereafter, multi-organ failure and death within little more than 24 hours, sometimes with a peculiar, greenish discolouration of the skin.

Lesser doses may be attended by no more than the oral reactions for some days. Then myocardial, hepatic and renal dysfunction may be revealed by electrocardiography and laboratory tests. Again these abnormalities tend to disappear on their own. But, after a few more days, lung changes make their appearance, with a reduction in the gas transfer factor and the presence of fine, diffuse opacities throughout the lung fields as seen on x-ray of the chest. These coincide with alveolar oedema, cellular infiltration and progressive fibrosis, which advances relentlessly until death takes place, 2-3 weeks later, by respiratory failure.

Diagnosis

With any case of suspected paraquat poisoning it is imperative to know at once whether the chemical has actually been swallowed. This can be shown by a positive blue colouration developing when 2 ml of 1 % sodium dithionate solution in normal sodium hydroxide is added to 10 ml of urine. A negative result is reassuring, but a positive finding does not necessarily imply a grave prognosis.

It is essential, then, to measure the level of paraquat in the blood, either by radioimmunoassay, or by gas chromatography. A nomogram has been constructed (see below) from which it can be deduced whether the patient's blood level falls below a line when a favourable outcome can be predicted, or above the line, when energetic treatment must be brought into action.

Treatment

Regardless of any vomiting that has taken place, gastric aspiration and lavage is advised and, after that, Fuller's Earth as a 30%

suspension, with magnesium sulphate 5%, to the extent of 250 ml should be left in the stomach. In this way, not only is the paraquat adsorbed, but the passage of the chemical-adsorbent complex through the gut is expedited. This dose can be repeated at 4-hourly intervals.

Alternatively, after the first instillation of adsorbent, whole gut irrigation should be instituted, with the massive water and electrolyte depletion so occasioned being made good.

Further withdrawal of the paraquat, which has already made its way into the body, may be to some extent accomplished by haemoperfusion, or by haemodialysis.

Unduly high levels of inspired oxygen should be withheld for as long as possible, for these seem to accentuate the lung damage.

The claims therapeutically for superoxide dismutase, together with d-propranolol, or for steroids and immunosuppressant drugs, have not been upheld. Unfortunately, it remains doubtful whether any of the current schemes of management, no matter how vigorously exercised, can be at all effective, except perhaps in borderline cases.

For diquat and morfamquat alone, clinical experience with overdoses is somewhat lacking, but the same attitude towards treatment is recommended.

Summary

- Poisoning by paraquat and related herbicides taken orally is a serious matter that demands immediate medical care.
- Whether or not to embark on active treatment is decided by urinary analysis or, more specifically, by measuring the levels of the chemical in the blood
- The stomach should be emptied promptly, adsorbents should be introduced into the gastrointestinal tract, the gut contents should be purged and haemodialysis, or haemoperfusion, should be applied

9.8 Nicotine

Today nicotine is used less often in agriculture than hitherto, but t still finds applications in horticulture, chiefly as a fumigant, when it may be inhaled.

Action

A dose orally of no more than 40 mg nicotine is said to be fatal for man. The action of this alkaloid is first to stimulate and then to depress all the autonomic ganglia throughout the body.

Signs and symptoms

As with smoking in the uninitiated so with direct nicotine exposure, nausea, dizziness, sweating, vomiting, salivation, hyperpnoea and tachycardia are all experienced. Cardiac arrhythmias, convulsions and death may soon follow.

Diagnosis

In practice this rests on the circumstances and history. Blood levels, although measurable, can be determined in only a few laboratories.

Treatment

There are no specific antidotes so, besides suppressing convulsions with injections of diazepam, management is entirely supportive.

Summary

- Acute nicotine poisoning can be very dangerous
- The symptoms resemble those from smoking in the uninitiated, but are much more accentuated
- Apart from controlling convulsions by means of diazepam injections, treatment is entirely non-specific and supportive

9.9 Rodenticides (see 9.10-9.13)

Chemicals for rat and mouse poisoning include:

- anticoagulants
- chloralose

- fluoroacetates
- phosphine

Their actions are very similar in both rodents and man.

9.10   Anticoagulants

These are based upon warfarin and related substances. The material is commonly supplied in concentrated form for dilution, so that the content of the baits as laid down for rodent control is customarily quite low. Rodent death is brought about by the animals repeatedly eating the chemical, whereby sooner or later they are rendered anticoagulant and succumb to uncontrolled bleeding, mostly internally.

Action

Anticoagulant rodenticides act in the same way as they do in man, interfering with the synthesis of certain blood-coagulating factors in the liver.

Signs and symptoms

Unless someone is so perverse as to devour an inordinate quantity of the concentrate, he is unlikely to be harmed. In round terms, more than 1 kg of bait would have to be eaten to render an adult, or child at risk.

Nevertheless, homicide has been contrived by the deliberate and repeated 'lacing' of food with anticoagulant concentrates.

Diagnosis

Proof of the diagnosis can be advanced by the finding of a prolonged prothrombin time in the blood.

Treatment

Only exceptionally will it be necessary to treat with vitamin K1.

9.11 Chloralose

In this rodenticide the active constituent is α-chloralose, a derivative of chloral hydrate.

Action

The chloral hydrate moiety which is released after uptake by the body is rapidly metabolised to trichlorethyl alcohol. This is a depressant to the central nervous system and may lead to death via coma and respiratory arrest.

Signs and symptoms

Whereas chloralose itself is a fairly powerful hypnotic, quite large quantities of the bait (popularly in a sponge cake base) would have to be eaten to make a human subject sleepy.

Diagnosis

Uncertainty about diagnosis can be dispelled by measuring the trichlorethanol concentration in the blood.

Treatment

This should be the same as for dealing with an overdose of chloral hydrate, or of barbiturates (see **8.6**).

9.12 Fluoroacetates

Fluoroacetates and fluoroacetamide are powerful, acute poisons of such toxicity that they are reserved for killing rodents in special situations, e.g. sewers and ships holds.

Action

In the mammalian body the fluoroacetates specifically block the tricarboxylic acid cycle of carbohydrate metabolism.

Signs and symptoms

These make their toxic presence felt within an hour or two after ingestion, with extreme anxiety, muscle twitchings, cardiac irregularities, convulsions, coma and collapse.

Diagnosis

Clinically there is no time to wait upon laboratory tests. It is possible to estimate blood fluoroacetate concentrations analytically, but the findings are of more use post-mortem.

Treatment

Beyond abating the convulsions with diazepam and injecting calcium gluconate intravenously, all that can be done is to maintain the respiration and offer supportive measures.

9.13   Phosphine

Phosphine in the gaseous state is highly toxic and does not lend itself to safe handling as a rodenticide. So, for the welfare of the operatives called upon to use it, preparations have been contrived to generate the gas on site. Aluminium phosphide, for example, can be formulated in the solid state and, with this, the ambient moisture can interact to produce phosphine, with its easily discernible fishy odour.

Action

Inhaled phosphine rapidly acts upon the central nervous and the gastrointestinal system.

Signs and symptoms

Abdominal pain and vomiting usually precede vertigo, ataxia, convulsions, coma and death.

Diagnosis

No laboratory tests are diagnostically informative.

Treatment

This can be little more than palliative.

9.14   Other pesticides

Among the other pesticides, arsenic and thallium are considered in more detail under sections **10.8** and **10.4** respectively. The remainder make up a miscellany with little in common between them toxicologically. Poisoning from them is seldom encountered in practice, they attract no specific, or antidotal, therapy and the management of patients exposed to them must be symptomatic and supportive. Only for gross, self-administered 2,4-D, a popular herbicide, is forced alkaline diuresis likely to be contemplated. Whenever there is ignorance about the nature and toxicity of any pesticide, the advice of a Poisons Information, or Poisons Control Service may be helpful, or a telephone call can sometimes be made to the manufacturer, or supplier, whose name, address and telephone number should be printed on the label.

9.15   Pesticide residues in food

Fears have often been expressed about the risks to ordinary members of the population from eating foodstuffs in which pesticide residues persist from treatment at some stage previously. So long as the chemicals have been applied at the recommended dose rates and in accordance with what is called 'good agricultural practice', these fears can be dismissed.

Very rarely, however, some mistake can be made whereby an excessive amount of one or other of these chemicals finds its way into the diet. The effect then on the consumer is the same as if the chemical had been directly ingested and treatment should be as for poisoning by the oral route.

9.0 Pesticides

Notes

9.0 Pesticides

Notes

9.0 Pesticides

Notes

10.0 Heavy metals and metalloids

10.0 Heavy metals and metalloids

10.0 Heavy metals and metalloids

10.1 Lead

These are grouped together more for editorial convenience than for their toxicological relationships. Further, with the individual metals, the toxicity differs according to the chemical compounds in which they are incorporated.

10.1 Lead

This metal abounds naturally, being distributed widely, if unevenly, throughout the earth's crust. It reaches the environment, or biosphere, by its recovery from natural deposits and its utilisation by man. In this way the community becomes exposed to it, virtually inescapably, in the atmosphere and in the diet, as well as by the uses to which it is put industrially. So long as this intake is balanced by excretion in the faeces and in the urine, man suffers no cumulation, but once the intake overtakes the elimination, the human body burden increases. Much of the element is then stored almost harmlessly in the bones. It is the excess in other tissues that exerts a more deleterious action.

Action

Lead that is free in the body enters into porphyrin metabolism and interferes with the normal synthesis of haem. It also acts upon the nervous system, centrally and peripherally.

Signs and symptoms

Truly acute poisoning from lead comes about only with certain salts of the metal, e.g. lead chloride. Then the toxicity is not strictly metallurgical, but is due to the ingested chemical behaving as an irritant upon the gastrointestinal mucosa, resulting in vomiting, diarrhoea and collapse. Metallic lead taken orally does not behave in this way.

Chronic poisoning from lead, environmentally or occupationally, may advance more subtly, symptoms appearing when the body load becomes excessive. This state is manifest by anorexia, a metallic taste in the mouth, constipation, cramping abdominal pain and peripheral nerve palsies, affecting the motor innervation and, more especially, that of the extensor groups of muscles. Inspection of the mouth may reveal a blue pigmented line along the gum margins (Burton's line).

10.0   Heavy metals and metalloids

10.1   Lead

Haematologically there is anaemia and punctate basophilia, while radiography of the bones may disclose a heightened density at the metaphyseal zones. If the lead has been ingested, discrete opacities may be seen radiographically in the gut, chiefly in the distal colon.

Severe cases may present as encephalopathy, above all in children, with headache, lassitude, irritability, raised intracranial pressure, convulsions and coma. It is alleged that even when the blood levels are within a range hitherto regarded as normal, lead may bring about intellectual impairment, again more so in children than in adults.

Poisoning from organic lead compounds declares itself predominantly by psychotic changes in the patient.

Diagnosis

Overt lead poisoning can be readily recognised by the symptom complex described above. Lesser grades of 'plumbism' can easily be overlooked unless laboratory tests are performed.

Normal people spared from undue exposure should have blood levels below 35 μg/100 ml (1.5 μmol l⁻¹). With figures higher than this, over-exposure should be suspected and findings above 80 μg/100 ml (4.0 μmol l⁻¹) are a signal for investigation and withdrawal of the person from any known further contact with lead. There is some reason to take this action at levels even of 60 μg/100 mg (3.0 μmol l⁻¹).

With frank lead poisoning, the concentrations in the blood may be much higher, though they are subject to considerable individual variation.

Supplementary laboratory tests for plumbism include amino laevulinic acid dehydratase (ALAD) in erythrocytes, amino laevulinic acid (ALA) in the urine and free erythrocyte protoporphyrin in the peripheral blood, but none of these is entirely specific for lead.

Treatment

Acute poisoning from soluble and irritant lead salts requires energetic supportive treatment to counteract the dehydration and loss of electrolytes.

Chronic poisoning merits specific, chelation therapy when there are overt symptoms and/or the blood lead levels are above 100 μg/100 ml (5.0 μmol l^{-1}) in adults and above 60-80 μg/100 ml (3.0-4.0 μmol l^{-1}) in children.

Having made sure that renal function is adequate and that there is a satisfactory output of urine, the following agents may be used:

Calcium disodium edetate (Ca-EDTA) is given at the rate, for an adult, of 50-75 mg kg^{-1} body weight daily for 5 days. This may be infused slowly by the intravenous route, each 2 g of the edetate being diluted with 250 ml normal saline, or it may be given in divided doses, 4-hourly, by deep intramuscular injection, along with procaine to lessen the pain. For children the dosage may be calculated on the basis of 1500 mg m^{-2} of body surface.

More effectively and in severe cases, notably those with encephalopathy, dimercaprol may be added as well. Over the first 2 days the dose of this agent for an adult should be 2.5-5.0 mg kg^{-1} body weight 4-hourly by deep, intramuscular injection or, for children, 80 mg m^{-2} body surface 4-hourly. If it is deemed advisable to prolong the course, the dose thereafter should be reduced to 2.5 mg kg^{-1} body weight twice-daily on the third day and 2.5 mg kg^{-1} body weight once on each of the fourth and fifth days.

Otherwise, in less serious cases, penicillamine orally may be used alone, at the rate of 250 mg to 2 g daily for an adult, or 600 mg m^{-2} body surface for a child, and this may be continued for some weeks, advisedly until the amount of lead voided in urine falls below 0.3 mg in 24 hours.

In principle, chelation therapy should not be withdrawn before the blood lead levels have been reduced to within the normal range, though it is not unusual for transient increases to be observed following cessation of such treatment.

For cerebral oedema, systemic corticosteroids may afford relief and fluid intake should be kept to an essential minimum. Attempts at surgical decompression are as fruitless as they are dangerous.

For *organic lead* poisoning the mental disturbances should be mitigated so far as possible by means of intravenous chlormethiazole, or by injections of chlorpromazine, with diazepam being added if convulsions obtrude. Only when the psychotic excesses have been controlled should chelation be embarked upon to dispose of the surfeit of lead from the body.

10.2 Mercury

Elemental mercury ('quicksilver'), if swallowed, has no action on the body, unless it is in a finely dispersed state, as it is in the old-fashioned purgative, 'grey powder', wherein the metal has been triturated with chalk. Then the minuscule droplets of the mercury react with the hydrochloric acid of the stomach to form the chloride, which is irritant to the gastrointestinal mucosa. On the other hand, when mercury comes into repeated contact with the skin it may be readily absorbed percutaneously to set up systemic 'hydrargism'. In other circumstances, metallic mercury may readily vaporise into the atmosphere and so be inhaled in quantities sufficient to bring about general, toxic effects.

Organic mercurial compounds, which have extensive usage as fungicides, can also reach the body via the skin, the lungs, or orally, so as to give rise to a distinctive symptom complex.

Action

Biochemically in the body the mercury ion seems to have an affinity for sulphydril bonds and so may disorganise the normal cellular metabolism, the nature of the resulting clinical disorder then depending on the anatomical site, in the various organs or tissues, at which these metabolic aberrations take place.

The mercuric salts, e.g. mercuric chloride, however, predominantly behave as tissue irritants and protein denaturants and so, in the gut, they bring about an acute enteritis which, in turn, may be followed by uptake of the mercury ion to induce systemic effects.

Signs and symptoms

When swallowed, the *inorganic mercurial salts* set up a 'burning' sensation in the mouth and throat, rapidly followed by vice-like pains substernally and in the epigastrium, with vomiting and devastating diarrhoea. The rapid depletion of fluid and electrolytes may precipitate cardiovascular collapse, along with proteinuria and renal failure.

Being odourless *mercury vapour* may be inhaled unwittingly in high concentrations, only to reveal itself a few hours later by a dry and distressing cough with dyspnoea, accompanied by pyrexia and pains in the muscles. Occasionally this acute phase gives way to renal damage and a raised excretion of mercury in the urine.

Breathing an atmosphere of *mercury vapour* in lower concentrations over a longer period may fail to provoke any acute reactions but, as with extended percutaneous exposure, it may nevertheless bring about chronic mercurial poisoning insidiously by cumulation of the metal in the body. This expresses itself as a metallic taste in the mouth, with personality changes, notably erethism, tiredness, mental depression, tremors, ataxia and intellectual disability.

Examination reveals stomatitis, gingivitis, and hypersalivation, with sometimes a blue, pigmented line at the gum margins (similar to that seen with lead) and 'mercurialentis' — a discolouration of the eyes seen when the lens is viewed with a slit-lamp.

The toxic action of the *organic mercurials* is centred upon the nervous system, with ataxia, involuntary movements and constriction of the visual fields. Pregnant women so afflicted may give birth to infants with severe congenital deformities.

Diagnosis

The clinical picture, coupled with the history, is nearly always sufficient to arrive at a diagnosis.

Mercury levels in the blood and urine can be measured by atomic absorption spectrophotometry, the normal maxima being 15 μg l^{-1} and 20 μg l^{-1} respectively. Higher concentrations are found with over-exposure, but the figures do not invariably correlate with the intensity of the poisoning clinically.

Treatment

Acute poisoning from *inorganic mercurial* salts calls for immediate, resuscitative management, with haemodialysis if renal failure supervenes. Thereafter, only when analytical findings point to an undue body load of mercury are there grounds for dimercaprol therapy.

With *metallic mercury*, the acute symptoms from inhalation respond to symptomatic measures. Where, however, the classical signs of chronic mercurial poisoning, either from inhalation or percutaneous uptake, are evident and the analytical figures are high, chelation should be undertaken with dimercaprol as for arsenic and with the same precautions (see **10.8**).

The psychological derangements brought about by *organic mercurials* call for anti-psychotic medication and care, with diazepam for convulsions. Chelation therapy is contraindicated.

In any form of hydrargism that leads to physical disability, rehabilitation may be required over a very long period.

10.3 Iron

Metallic iron itself raises no problem of toxicity, though there are individuals with inborn errors of metabolism, i.e. haemochromatosis, for whom iron behaves as a chronic systemic poison.

Iron salts (e.g. ferrous sulphate, ferrous gluconate, ferrous succinate, etc.) are formulated pharmaceutically for the treatment of anaemia. In acute overdose these can be very dangerous, particularly in children.

Action

Taken orally the iron salts are gastrointestinal irritants. The integrity of the gut mucosa selectively to transfer iron to the body is then deranged, so that iron may be absorbed to excess and so cause injury, principally to the brain and the liver.

Signs and symptoms

Within a few hours of taking an excess of iron salts by mouth there is epigastric pain, vomiting, haematemesis and diarrhoea. At this early stage there may be circulatory collapse. Then, after an illusory interval of recovery, the secondary symptom complex emerges, with encephalitis, pulmonary oedema, metabolic acidosis, renal failure and further collapse. Survival after this stage may be jeopardised by hepatic failure.

Diagnosis

Apart from the signs and history, a serum iron level above 8 mg l^{-1} (145 μmol l^{-1}) in an adult, or 5 mg l^{-1} (90 μmol l^{-1}) in a child portends dangerous poisoning.

Treatment

Once it has been decided that the iron poisoning is of serious intensity gastric lavage should be performed using a solution of desferrioxamine (2 g in 1 litre water), after which 2 g desferrioxamine in 10 ml sterile water should be left in the stomach. As soon as possible another 2 g of this agent should be injected intramuscularly, followed by a slow, intravenous infusion at the rate of 15 mg kg^{-1} body weight per hour, up to a total of 80 mg kg^{-1} in 24 hours.

Simultaneously, energetic resuscitation should be applied, with emphasis on restoring the fluid and electrolyte loss so as to protect against cardiovascular collapse. Renal failure is a signal for peritoneal dialysis, or haemodialysis, not only to obviate the excretory inadequacy, but also to provide an outlet for the chelated iron.

Encephalopathy is managed symptomatically. Intracranial decompression surgically for cerebral oedema is disappointing. Liver failure is also dealt with conservatively. After the heroic acute stages have been relieved, there may still be stenotic complications in the gut, due to enteric cicatrisation in the wake of necrosis, and these may call for surgery.

10.4   Thallium

Widely utilised though it is in industry, thallium does not seem to create any occupational hazards thereby. Moreover, as a personal depilatory, it has lost favour over recent years. In some countries, however, thallium salts are still employed as rodenticides and ant-killers, and being accessible in this way, they can be swallowed, accidentally or deliberately, with alarmingly toxic consequences. More sinisterly, from time to time thallium sulphate is still the selected agent for homicidal excursions.

Action

The biochemical mode of action of thallium is still not understood and all that can be said is that its metabolism is related to that of potassium. Little more than 1 gram by mouth can be fatal for man.

Signs and symptoms

After a single dose of a thallium salt, such as the sulphate, there is, to begin with, such a mild gastroenteritic reaction that it may pass unnoticed. For a day or two thereafter the patient may go about passably well, albeit admitting to general weakness. Then there may be complaint of 'burning' sensations in the extremities, chiefly in the soles of the feet and the palms of the hands, together with muscle weakness, ataxia and constipation. Moderate, bilateral ptosis may be noticed. Later comes a progressive polyneuritis, with insomnia and psychotic changes, which are apt to be dismissed as hysterical. Tachycardia heralds toxic myocarditis. Later still the almost pathognomic alopecia becomes apparent, this being preceeded, on careful scrutiny, by black pigmentation at the roots of the hairs.

The clinical recognition of thallium poisoning is probably more often overlooked than any other acutely toxic event.

Diagnosis

In the presence of thallium poisoning, analysis of the blood and urine shows levels markedly above 10 μg l^{-1} and 20 μg l^{-1} respectively. (The metal is not a normal constituent of the body.)

Treatment

Untreated, thallium poisoning can easily be fatal, for the acute lethal dose of the sulphate salt is so small.

Once the diagnosis is clear, the specific antidote potassium ferrihexacyanate (Berlin (Prussian) Blue) should be given via a stomach tube or, preferably, via an intraduodenal tube in twice daily doses of 10 g, together with magnesium sulphate as a purge. This chelates the thallium within the gut, so that it is excreted in the faeces and is not absorbed. That metal which has already penetrated to the tissues is regarded as beyond reach of the antidote, though it is usually advocated that the chelation should be maintained until the blood and urine levels of thallium return to normal. More often, chelation is discontinued when the metal can no longer be detected in the faeces. Otherwise, only symptomatic treatment is feasible.

Summary

- Early diagnosis is critical to the satisfactory management of cases of thallium poisoning, for in clinical toxicology, this is more commonly missed than any other aetiology.
- In effect, the specific antidote here, potassium ferrihexacyanate (Prussian Blue; Berlin Blue), is intended to inhibit uptake from the gut to the body systematically, for once this metal reaches the tissues, little can be done to suppress its toxic action.

10.5 Copper

Copper is found widely in nature and is an essential element to most forms of life, but the margin between the vital requirements and toxic levels is a narrow one. In the familial, metabolic disorder known as Wilson's disease, copper accumulates in the body, leading to hepatolenticular degeneration.

Action

Apart from Wilson's disease and possibly analogous pathologies, metallic copper is not toxic in practice. Physiologically it may be involved with iron metabolism.

The soluble salts, e.g. copper sulphate, can be corrosive towards living tissues, however, and a single dose of about 10 g orally can be fatal to man.

Signs and symptoms

Ingestion of copper sulphate and allied salts results in acute gastroenteritis, which can be extreme enough for cardiovascular collapse to ensue. Excess copper may then be absorbed to bring about intravascular haemolysis.

Diagnosis

There is no place for analytical investigations in this type of poisoning except, perhaps, post-mortem. Circumstances dictate therapy.

Treatment

This is directed at strenuous resuscitation, with replacement blood transfusion if haemolysis warrants it.

10.6 Lithium

This is another metal that, today, enjoys wide and diverse use in industry.

Lithium carbonate is prescribed medically for the amelioration of manic-depressive illness.

Action

Biochemically the action of lithium has not been truly elucidated, but it may have intracellular interactions with sodium and potassium and it undoubtedly modifies the renal excretion of these ions.

Signs and symptoms

These are seen most often when lithium accumulates from repeated therapeutic dosing with the carbonate, rather than from acute overdose. Symptoms include drowsiness, excessive thirst, polyuria, diarrhoea, mental retardation and convulsions. Increased muscular tone and brisk tendon reflexes are found on examination, while protein may be detected in the urine.

The hydride of lithium is highly corrosive.

Diagnosis

Blood level estimations are confirmatory, with normal levels for lithium being less than $1.30 \, \mu mol \, l^{-1}$, though patients vary considerably in their response to higher concentrations.

Treatment

This is primarily supportive, with resort to diazepam for convulsions. While the urinary excretion of lithium can be accelerated by forced alkaline diuresis, this may easily put the patient in peril from derangement of the sodium-potassium balance. Peritoneal dialysis, or haemodialysis, is likely to be safer and more effective.

Summary

* Lithium poisoning commonly arises from therapeutic overdose
* The symptoms include drowsiness, thirst, polyuria, mental changes and convulsions
* The diagnosis can be confirmed by measuring the blood lithium level
* Treatment is supportive, with peritoneal dialysis, or haemodialysis, in severe cases

10.7   Other metals

Numerous other metals may be of toxic consequence occupationally, e.g. antimony, barium, beryllium, chromium, manganese, nickel, tin, etc., and for the relevant information it is suggested that more specialist texts be consulted.

Suffice here to mention that soluble zinc salts resemble those of copper in their action on the gut and the fumes of zinc, characteristically associated with copper in brass, may be responsible for metal fume fever ('brass founder's ague'), an acute self-limiting condition that resembles influenza.

The fumes of cadmium, too, may appear innocent enough, but a quite transient exposure to high concentrations, especially from heating contaminated solder ('silver solder'), may set up a fulminating illness some hours later that, again, may be misdiagnosed as influenza, with cough, pyrexia and myalgia, but which may also proceed to acute pulmonary oedema and respiratory insufficiency, rapidly proving fatal. Renal damage may occur as well. Treatment, again, is only palliative and attempts at chelation may make matters worse.

The insoluble barium salts, e.g. barium sulphate, as used in contrast radiography, may be harmless enough, but their soluble counterparts, e.g. barium chloride, if swallowed, set up acute gastroenteritis, with weakness, paralysis of the skeletal muscles, convulsions and toxic myocarditis. Treatment is confined to symptomatic relief.

Summary

- Among the metals encountered industrially volatile zinc can be responsible for an influenza-like illness — metal fume fever, which is not serious and which is self-limiting
- Cadmium fumes are much more dangerous, for following an influenza-like illness, there may be pulmonary oedema, renal damage and sudden death
- Barium salts are toxic when swallowed only if they are soluble, e.g. barium chloride, as distinct from barium sulphate, the latter being used in contrast radiography

10.8   Arsenic

Even if arsenic, strictly speaking, is not a metal, but a metalloid, it is conveniently described in this section. The element is found widely distributed in nature, sometimes in undue abundance, as it does in certain areas of the Andes where the community suffers from endemic, arsenical poisoning in consequence. Prolonged exposure, moreover, is conducive to cancer.

Arsenicals are used in industry, as pesticides, in medicaments, and are still exploited homicidally.

Whereas chronic arsenical poisoning is still not exceptional today, the acute form is seldom seen. Chronic arsenicalism may be due to oral or percutaneous uptake. Acute reactions to arsenic, either accidental or deliberate (and homicide can still be perpetrated), are usually attributable to the swallowing of soluble arsenicals, of which arsenic trioxide is still the principal example. The picture of acute poisoning, without the characteristic enteric symptoms, can nevertheless be traced to other channels of entry as, for example, the packing of the vagina repeatedly with organic arsenicals in excessive doses.

Action

In the tissues arsenic is said to bind with sulphydril enzyme systems. The trivalent compounds, for which the fatal dose for man can be as little as 100 mg, are more toxic than the penta-valent compounds, and the organic arsenicals are less toxic still.

Signs and symptoms

Acute arsenical poisoning is typically illustrated when arsenic trioxide is swallowed. A rough gritty taste may be noticed in the mouth but, thereafter, nothing alarming may apparently happen for an hour or two, when there is precipitate vomiting and choleraic diarrhoea with abdominal pain, quickly predisposing to dehydration, electrolyte depletion and cardiovascular collapse. A decreased urine flow and proteinuria may be found and, at the same time, cardiac irregularities may intrude.

Chronic arsenical poisoning, from modest ingestion of perhaps a fortified food or drink, or a pharmaceutical 'tonic', or exposure occupationally over a period of time, may be insufficient to declare itself by any acute manifestations but may eventually attract attention on account of anorexia, mild but recurrent diar-rhoea and weight loss, that can be mistaken at first for 'asthenia'. Then comes the so-called 'raindrop' pattern on the skin, hyper-keratosis of the palms of the hands and soles of the feet, together with thickening of the nails and peripheral neuritis, all of which should leave the diagnosis no longer in doubt.

Diagnosis

Treatment of *acute* arsenical poisoning cannot be deferred for laboratory investigations. Yet it is wise to retain specimens of vomitus, faeces and urine for analysis later, if only for forensic reasons.

10.8 Arsenic

In *chronic* poisoning the preferred specimens for analysis are those of nail-clippings, or better still, hair withdrawn by the roots. These are then subjected to neutron activation. Concentrations of arsenic can then be explicitly expressed in relation to 1 mm lengths of hair, which not only point to the intensity of the poisoning, but also, since the hair grows at a fairly regular rate and the element is deposited sequentially therein, allows the exposure to be dated.

Treatment

Acute arsenical poisoning constitutes an emergency, for which prompt and vigorous resuscitative and supportive treatment is obligatory. The fluid and electrolyte depletion should be restored immediately, for this is the keystone to successful therapy. Nevertheless, *dimercaprol* as the specific antidote should be given as well, the dose being 2.5-5.0 mg kg^{-1} body weight, by deep intramuscular injection. Over the first 24 hours or, better still, over the first two days, this should be repeated at 4-hourly intervals, thereafter reducing the dose to 2.5 mg kg^{-1} body weight twice daily and not discontinuing until the patient has:

1 Fully recovered clinically, or
2 The plasma levels of arsenic have returned to normal, or
3 The total duration of this antidotal therapy has extended over 8 days.

For chronic arsenical poisoning, the source of exposure should be traced and, at once, withdrawn, taking note meanwhile of any suspicious circumstances. Then, the excess of arsenic in the body should be disposed of by dimercaprol chelation, in accordance with the schedule described above, and until urinary arsenic levels return to normal.

Symptomatic treatment may be required as well.

Summary

- Acute arsenical poisoning usually comes about from swallowing soluble arsenical compounds
- Chronic arsenical poisoning can arise from the repeated libations of 'tonics' containing arsenic, from wilful fortifying of food and drink, or from occupational exposure

- Gastrointestinal symptoms are prominent, with vomiting, diarrhoea, dehydration and collapse. In chronic arsenical poisoning, 'rain-drop' pigmentation of the skin and peripheral neuritis are seen
- Treatment is primarily supportive, coupled with dimercaprol as the specific antidote
- Analytical confirmation of the diagnosis is helpful

10.9 Arsine

Arsine (A_2H_3), an arsenical derivative, is a gas which is either handled in the pure state in industry, hopefully with the essential precautions to protect workers, or it is liberated adventitiously and unexpectedly from other metals contaminated with this element whenever they come into contact with nascent hydrogen. This latter situation can easily arise when, for example, metal parts are dipped in acid, or metallic dross is sprayed with hot water. Industrial accidents of this type occur too often, even now.

Action

Arsine has the singular property of haemolysing the mature erythrocytes by a mechanism that remains obscure. Haemopoiesis, as such, is unaffected.

Signs and symptoms

Even in remarkably low concentrations, inhaled arsine makes its way rapidly into the blood stream via the lungs. The resulting clinical picture is the outcome of the haemolysis to which it then gives rise.

There is malaise, abdominal pain and vomiting, while the patient usually notices red-brown discolouration of the urine. The conjuctivae take on a coppery-red tone, and generalised jaundice, together with anaemia, makes its appearance a day or so later. In severe cases, pulmonary oedema develops and the patient becomes comatose.

Death at this stage is usually referable to toxic myocarditis and cardiac failure.

Delirium and renal failure, with haemoglobinuria, are commonly seen in the absence of an early, fatal outcome. Sometimes there is liver damage as well.

Diagnosis

This can nearly always be substantiated by the history, and the symptoms and signs as outlined above. Arsenic measurements in the blood and other tissues are seldom of more than retrospective value.

Treatment

Replacement blood transfusion should be commenced at once, with haemodialysis if renal failure should complicate the condition. Liver damage should be managed conservatively.

Summary

- Arsine gas, which may be liberated industrially without being recognised from some metals and dross, can be highly toxic if inhaled
- It leads to acute haemolysis and renal damage
- Treatment is by exchange blood transfusion and haemodialysis

10.0 Heavy metals and metalloids

Notes

10.0 Heavy metals and metalloids

Notes

11.0 Industrial gases, fumigants, etc.

11.0 Industrial gases, fumigants, etc.

Numerous gases, fumigants and volatile solvents are employed in industry and, to some extent they are met with in every day life. Individually they vary enormously in their physicochemical characteristics and in their toxicity. Few medical experts are conversant with all of them, with their dangers and with the treatment of human exposure. Certain general principles can nevertheless be enunciated for the management of emergencies arising therefrom.

11.1 First aid

Whenever someone is thought to be overcome by a gas or a vapour, the clamant necessity is to remove the victim from the contaminated atmosphere, with the rescuers taking care not to endanger themselves in so doing. Where vapour inhalation can be traced to volatile liquids splashed on the clothing, this should be removed at once and the skin washed, preferably by some form of showering. As asphyxia is always a likelihood, a clear airway should be ensured and precautions taken against ventilatory failure. Removal of the patient to hospital should be arranged at the earliest moment, resuscitation being maintained *en route*.

11.2 Hospital care

For few cases of inhalation poisoning are specific measures applicable. Hospital care must therefore be supportive, with particular regard to the respiratory system, without neglecting the cardiovascular system and the fluid balance meanwhile. If pulmonary oedema should develop, mechanical ventilation, with positive, end-expiratory pressure (PEEP), is essential. Diuretics achieve little in dispersing the oedema that accumulates in this way.

11.3 Methane; natural gas

Unlike 'town gas' (coal gas), methane does not bring about carboxyhaemoglobinaemia, but asphyxiation. The greater hazard is of fire and explosion

Treatment is that for asphyxia, with oxygen and respiratory support.

11.4 Petroleum products

These are, in the main, aliphatic hydrocarbons which may embody a modicum of aromatic hydrocarbons (even benzene in traces) as well. Most commercial petrol has contained, as an additive, a small percentage of organic lead as an 'anti-knock' agent.

Signs and symptoms

When swallowed, these petroleum products exert a low intrinsic toxicity and it is best to avoid purposeful emptying of the stomach for fear of bronchial aspiration. Spontaneous vomiting in itself can bring about this complication. Emphasis should therefore be placed on care of the lungs and the management of any bronchopneumonic sequelae.

Repeated skin contact, by a defatting action, can predispose sometimes to a contact dermatitis.

Inhaled petrol and similar vapours may be responsible for progressive dizziness, incoordination, ataxia and loss of consciousness, with or without convulsions. There is said to be a risk occasionally of sensitisation of the myocardium.

Treatment

Treatment should be supportive, with special regard to cardiac dysrhythmias and acute cardiac failure.

Chronic exposure to hydrocarbon products containing benzene (and more so, of course, to benzene itself) may predispose to leukopenia and anaemia of the aplastic type. Every care should therefore be taken to avoid this by suitable occupational hygiene, but once the blood dyscrasia becomes established it requires fresh blood transfusions and energetic haematological support.

11.5 Chlorinated hydrocarbons

Among this group of chemical compounds, carbon tetrachloride is the toxicological prototype. Chloroform is similar. Tetrachloroethylene (perchlorethylene) and other derivatives, which have largely superseded carbon tetrachloride as cleaning agents, are much less hazardous.

Signs and symptoms

Besides the usual features of narcosis, mimicking inhalation anaesthesia, along with respiratory depression, there may be some cerebral excitation. More ominously, cardiac arrhythmias may arise, and gastrointestinal symptoms that proceed to acute hepatic failure, especially if alcohol (ethanol) is taken at the same time. The hepatic damage may be delayed in onset for a few days, but it can occur from a relatively minor exposure, bringing in its train renal dysfunction.

Treatment

Again the principles of supportive management apply, with respiratory maintenance taking priority, followed by the conventional methods for dealing with liver and kidney failure, if these complications should aggravate the condition of the patient.

11.6 Fluorinated hydrocarbons

These are widely encountered as propellants in aerosols. Toxicologically they are akin to the chlorinated hydrocarbons and, from excessive inhalation, there is a possibility of cardiac arrhythmias and acute cardiac failure. Treatment is supportive and symptomatic.

11.7 Fumigants

Carbon tetrachloride, to which reference has already been made, still finds some use as a commercial fumigant, but it should be handled with meticulous care so that workers are protected from the effects on the central nervous system, the liver and the kidney.

Ethylene dichloride

As a pesticide fumigant, ethylene dichloride is today less widely employed than hitherto on account of the suspicion that it may be carcinogenic. The acute reactions from inhalation are those of unsteadiness and ataxia, seldom proceeding to loss of consciousness. Treatment is according to symptoms.

Ethylene dibromide

Like the dichloride, ethylene dibromide looks as though it is being phased out as a fumigant, in the belief that by long-term exposure it is carcinogenic.

Locally it behaves as an irritant. There is little to fear from acute inhalation, though subsequent liver damage has been reported.

Methyl bromide

This is a volatile liquid which, as a vapour in the atmosphere at a concentration above about 1 %, can be detected by its smell and irritant properties.

Actions
These are not clearly understood, though some interaction would appear to take place with protein molecules.

Signs and symptoms
Topically methyl bromide liquid is a strong vesicant, and, on the skin, it causes itching and blistering, usually after an interval of an hour-or-so. Similarly the vapour is very irritating towards the eyes and the mucosae.

Inhalation gives rise to headache, visual disturbance, ataxia, weakness, peripheral paraesthesia and sometimes convulsions and renal damage. High concentrations can induce coma and pulmonary oedema.

Diagnosis
Recognition of acute methyl bromide poisoning is usually obvious from the history and circumstances.

Over-exposure in the absence of symptoms can be revealed by measuring the levels of blood bromide, preferably in the organic form, and regular workers with this fumigant are advisedly monitored in this way.

Treatment
Few textile, or rubber-type, materials afford satisfactory protection against methyl bromide. Soiled clothing should, therefore, be removed, contaminated skin should be washed and any dermal lesions should be treated symptomatically.

Whenever the gas has been inhaled the patient should be kept under observation for at least 48 hours. Pulmonary oedema can develop suddenly; it should be treated in the normal manner and with systemic corticosteroids. Renal damage may be such as to require haemodialysis.

Organic disorders of the central nervous system respond to palliative measures, though psychological symptoms may persist for some time after all the physical signs have disappeared.

11.8 Chloropicrin

This may be added to other fumigants as a warning agent.

Action

In the presence of water, chloropicrin decomposes to hydrochloric acid, nitric acid and carbon dioxide, and under the influence of light it may be converted, in small measure, to phosgene.

Signs and symptoms

On the skin and eyes chloropicrin is an intense irritant and, when inhaled, bronchospasm and pulmonary oedema may develop.

Treatment

This is entirely symptomatic.

It is an irritant with a distinctively unpleasant odour ('bad eggs'). Nevertheless, despite these warning attributes, poisoning may overcome a person before evasive retreat may be taken.

Unfortunately, no antidote treatment corresponding to that for cyanide poisoning has yet been devised, so only symptomatic measures can be offered, not forgetting to take immediate steps to remove the victim from further exposure.

11.9 Formaldehyde (formalin)

Formaldehyde is a gas which readily dissolves in water to yield formalin solution. This chemical has found well-nigh universal employment as a disinfectant, fumigant and preservative. It is also involved with air pollution.

Signs and symptoms

In the atmosphere formaldehyde gas is highly irritant, causing lachrymation, soreness of the eyes, coughing, dyspnoea, bronchial irritation and pulmonary oedema.

If formalin is swallowed it behaves as a corrosive (see **12.0**) as does its polymer, the solid metaldehyde, which is widely used as a slug bait.

Treatment

Reactions to the vapour should be treated symptomatically, having made certain that the patient is withdrawn from further exposure. When formalin, or metaldehyde is swallowed, the treatment is the same as for corrosive poisoning (see **12.4**).

11.10 Phosgene

This gas owes its notoriety to its place in warfare. It can also be a hazard occupationally in certain industries. Said to possess a 'geranium'-like odour, its treachery relates to the symptom-free hours that can elapse between exposure and the unexpected onset of often overwhelming pulmonary oedema that is disposed only to symptomatic relief.

11.11 Summary of gases

- Some industrial gases are simply asphyxiants, some are narcotic, others are irritant as well. In addition, some vapours, e.g. carbon tetrachloride, are hepatotoxic, others, e.g. fluorinated hydrocarbons, are sensitising to the myocardium and others still, e.g. methyl bromide, can bring about multiple organ damage

- The first step is always to remove the victim from the contaminated atmosphere and prevent further exposure
- Next, adequate oxygen and ventilation should be assured
- Finally, careful observation should be maintained for any other abnormalities which should promptly be treated symptomatically and supportively

11.12   Cyanides

Cyanides retain a prominent place as pesticides, but it is not by such use alone that poisoning may arise. They enter into a number of industrial processes, e.g. silver plating, so that occupational exposure is a hazard always to be reckoned with.

Inorganic cyanides, such as those of sodium and potassium, are highly toxic if swallowed, less than 0.5 g by mouth being fatal for man. These salts may also be absorbed percutaneously. Even more dangerous, though, is hydrogen cyanide gas, which on inhalation can be hazardous in quite low concentrations. It has the odour of bitter almonds, but this is not readily detectable by everyone.

Another source of cyanide is to be found within the kernels of some fruits, such as apricot and almond, in which it exists in an organically bound form, amygdalin. It does so in laetrile, which has been promoted as an unorthodox anticancer drug. Within the gut the cyanogenic amygdalin, which is in itself harmless, may be broken down by the intestinal flora to release the toxic cyanide moiety.

Action

Biochemically the mode of action of cyanide is quite specific. It blocks cytochrome oxidase, so that oxidative metabolism and phosphorylation are brought to a halt. In spite, therefore, of high peripheral oxygen tensions and a surfeit of oxyhaemoglobin, the cells are starved of available oxygen; hence the term 'histotoxic hypoxia'.

169

11.12   Cyanides

Signs and symptoms

These may appear promptly after the inhalation of hydrogen cyanide, and rapidly, or after a delay of a few hours, when cyanide has been swallowed (depending on the state, or fullness, of the stomach). The interval is longer still when the offending material is organically bound.

The subject is first aware of a sensation of dizziness and alarm, succeeded by headache, tachycardia and a constrictive feeling in the chest. Because of the directly stimulant action of cyanide upon the chemoreceptors, hyperpnoea develops, and there is confusion, ataxia, weakness, vertigo, disorientation and collapse. Death is by respiratory arrest.

Cyanosis is absent and the skin and mucosae may display a distinctly 'cherry red' colouration.

Diagnosis

Blood levels of cyanide may be measured, but there is no time for such procrastination in the face of acute poisoning. Urgent treatment is paramount. Specimens may nevertheless be collected later for medico-legal reference.

Treatment

As a first-aid measure a capsule of amyl nitrite should be broken under the patient's nose so that the volatile contents may be inhaled, meanwhile making sure that he is ventilating — though eschewing the mouth-to-mouth method of artificial respiration. This manoeuvre can be repeated at intervals of a few minutes.

Treatment with dicobalt edetate is more effective. Ordinarily this is innocuous, though sometimes it may induce severe tachycardia, hypotension and chest pain, the more so if the original diagnosis was wrong, or the exposure was so mild as not to merit the antidote. For these reasons — despite the emergency otherwise — the cobalt edetate should be withheld unless the patient evinces unmistakable signs of poisoning.

A solution of 300-600 mg *dicobalt edate* (Kelocyanor) should be injected intravenously over the course of a few minutes. If there is no obvious benefit from this, a further 300 mg should be given, with oxygen and support to the ventilation. Lack of response should infer misdiagnosis and then there is no point in persisting with the antidote.

An alternative treatment for cyanide poisoning is the injection intravenously, first of 10 ml of 3 % sterile solution of *sodium nitrate* over a few minutes and then a similar slow injection of 25 ml of a 50 % sterile solution of *sodium thiosulphate.*

Neutralising mixtures, as e.g. of sodium carbonate and ferrous carbonate, to be given orally in cases of cyanide poisoning by mouth are often suggested, but they must be freshly prepared, are not very feasible and are of doubtful value. Gastric aspiration and lavage may nevertheless recover significant amounts of any cyanide recently swallowed, but the manoeuvre needs to be performed with uncommon alacrity.

In acute poisoning, attempts at measuring the blood levels of cyanide are tantamount to disregarding the patient's welfare in deference to scientific curiosity.

Ventilation of the lungs should be safeguarded throughout, metabolic acidosis should be corrected, and any patient adversely affected should be kept at rest for a few days during which a check should be made on any anoxic, myocardial damage that may have occurred.

Summary

- Acute cyanide poisoning is a critical medical emergency recognised from the patient's history of exposure
- In the first-aid situation repeated inhalations of amyl nitrite should be given
- Once symptoms such as dizziness, headache, tightness of the chest, palpitations and dyspnoea appear, the specific antidote, dicobalt edetate (Kelocyanor) should be injected intravenously at a dose of 300-600 mg over the course of a few minutes
- Ventilation of the lungs should be maintained, but not by the mouth-to-mouth technique.

11.13   Hydrogen sulphide

This gas is mentioned here, first, because it is an occupational
hazard in certain locations, notably sewers, and second because
its toxic mode of action is analogous to that of cyanide. Its
effects, however, are not reversed by cobalt edetate, or other
cyanide antidotes, and treatment, therefore, is solely supportive.

11.0 Industrial gases, fumigants, etc.

Notes

11.0 Industrial gases, fumigants, etc.

Notes

12.0 Irritants, corrosives and caustics

12.0 Irritants, corrosives and caustics

12.1 Action / 12.2 Signs and symptoms

In the world today there must be in circulation a host of chemicals that are variously irritant, corrosive or caustic to living tissues, with a potential for damaging the skin and mucosae topically and for eroding the gut if swallowed. Against this background it is remarkable how relatively few incidents of this kind, of any severity, in fact assail the human population. Accidents can nevertheless overtake adults and, to a greater degree, small children who do not appreciate the horrors associated with such materials. Moreover some individuals, although perhaps fewer than in the past, turn to these unpleasant chemicals as a means of suicide.

12.1 Action

Irritants and corrosives are basically protein-coagulants which thereby bring about the necrosis of living cells. Caustics or alkalis have the same action, but they tend to be more destructive.

12.2 Signs and symptoms

Directly applied to the skin, these chemicals produce painful reddening, inflammation, blistering, ulceration or even penetrating necrosis. Their effects on the eye, or on the mucosae, are the same.

Often the damage is confined to the site of contact, but sometimes by rupturing the integrity of the skin, or other surfaces, they provide a portal of entry for systemic uptake.

When swallowed, there is physicochemical trauma to the upper gastrointestinal tract, with denudation of the mucosal lining and sometimes penetration to, or even through, the muscular layer, with a likelihood of perforation. The mouth and pharynx are the initial targets for this assault but, strangely enough, these regions may exceptionally be almost spared, whereas the larynx may be eroded, or become oedematous, so compromising respiration, or the oesophagus and stomach may bear the brunt of the attack. Once more, systemic absorption may be a secondary phenomenon.

To begin with the patient is stricken with a burning, throttling sensation in the mouth and throat, associated with strenuous retching. Then there is a sharp, dagger-like pain in the chest substernally, followed by searing, epigastric pain and vomiting, sometimes with haematemesis. Dysphagia soon becomes established. Staining and excoriation, from spilling or rejection, may be observed circumorally and down the chin.

Generalised collapse may supervene and perforation of the oesophagus or stomach is always a possibility. Survival from the acute stage may be compromised by cicatrical stenosis of the alimentary tract and consequential gut obstruction.

No more than 10-20 ml of concentrated hydrochloric, sulphuric, nitric, oxalic, or formic acid, or the corresponding volumes of concentrated caustic solutions, may prove fatal by mouth.

12.3 Diagnosis

This is usually obvious from the circumstances and appearances. Confirmatory tests are neither pertinent, nor necessary.

12.4 Treatment

The perils of gastric aspiration and lavage outweigh any possible advantages, while attempts at neutralisation, by administering bases for acids, and weak acids (e.g. vinegar) for caustics, are utterly misplaced.

Milk or water may be given by mouth as a diluent, providing the swallowing reflex is intact. Where pain is distressing, injections of an opiate analgesic afford much-needed relief.

The airway must be preserved, either by an endotracheal catheter, or even by tracheostomy, and respiratory care may be needed for bronchial aspiration.

Cardiovascular collapse must be countered by a rigorous supportive regime, with the replacement of fluids and electrolytes.

Ongoing observation should not be relaxed, for with signs of perforation, surgical intervention is mandatory.

12.0 Irritants, corrosives and caustics

12.4 Treatment

Some medical authorities urge endoscopy when, in the absence of arresting signs in the mouth or throat, it may still be possible to reveal trauma in the oesophagus or stomach. Others would inveigh against this manoeuvre as a routine, putting reliance rather on clinical appraisal. Likewise, there is no unanimity about the value of giving systemic corticosteroids to lessen the cicatrisation that brings about stenosis.

Whilst sharing the undesirable toxicity of the other corrosives, *formic acid*, which still figures in many homes as a kettle-descaler, or bath cleaner, can be absorbed by the body so as to cause systemic acidosis, haematuria and renal damage. The acidosis must be corrected by infusions intravenously of sodium bicarbonate and any renal failure circumvented by haemodialysis.

Likewise, *oxalic acid* and *hydrofluoric acid*, the latter being a vicious corrosive, can obtain access to the body from the gut and therein react with calcium, depleting these ions, so that tetany and convulsions are induced. For this condition, 10 % calcium gluconate should be given intravenously and repeated as indicated. With the oxalic acid, too, there is a possibility of oxalate being deposited in the kidneys and causing renal damage.

When inhaled, moreover, *hydrogen fluoride* is intensely irritating to the respiratory tract and demands oxygen, bronchial toilet and preservation of ventilation.

The skin burns from acids and alkalis should be treated by liberal irrigation with saline, or water, and then by dressing as for thermal burns. If the desquamation is extensive, skin grafting may be indicated later. For hydrofluoric acid burns, which can be excessively painful as well as penetrating, irrigation should be followed by subcutaneous injection with a 10 % calcium gluconate solution, or the application of calcium gluconate gel. In severe cases, direct regional intra-arterial infusion of 10-20 ml of 20 % calcium gluconate solution in normal saline may be called for.

Any contact of acids or alkalis with the eyes should be regarded as of grave import. Immediate irrigation is required. This is more easily urged than achieved, above all in the home, workplace or field. The eye must be kept open during the manoeuvre, for a small flushing of the cornea and conjunctiva achieves far more than a voluminous washing circumorbitally. Pain may be relieved by the instillation of local anaesthetic drops. Where solid patches of lime reach the eye and become embedded they must be removed physically.

In any event, after first aid treatment, anyone who has suffered from corrosive, or caustic, injury to the eye should be referred for expert ophthalmic assessment.

12.5   Phenol

At one time an almost ubiquitous disinfectant in so many homes, phenol today has been largely supplanted by less toxic substitutes. When it is swallowed, comes into contact with the skin and mucosae, or finds its way into the eye, it acts as a corrosive and should be treated accordingly. If ingested, olive oil, or a similar vegetable oil by mouth will prove both soothing and inhibitory to absorption from the gut.

Phenol is peculiar, however, in so far as it gives rise to surprisingly little pain, because it destroys the peripheral afferent nerve endings. More seriously, it is rapidly absorbed from the gastrointestinal tract, or through the skin, to set up systemic phenol poisoning, with convulsions, coma, respiratory depression, haemolysis and methaemoglobineamia, discolouration of the urine with haemoglobinuria and renal damage. General, supportive management is called for and, initially, diuresis, though renal failure may necessitate haemodialysis. Rarely is the methaemoglobinaemia of such severity as to warrant giving methylene blue intravenously.

12.6   Methylene chloride (dichloromethane)

Nowadays, with a vogue for paint-stripping chemically in preference to physically, methylene chloride is the principal constituent of many products marketed industrially and domestically for this purpose. Children have died from inadvertently drinking proprietory paint-strippers. When methylene chloride is swallowed, or gets on to the skin, or into the eyes, it should be treated as for any other corrosive. In addition, though, its systemic absorption is demonstrated by dizziness, bronchopneumonia, toxic mycocarditis and haemolysis, all of which should be treated conservatively.

Exposure to methylene chloride vapour in an enclosed atmosphere can result in methaemoglobinaemia, which can intensify the cardiac insufficiency in anyone so disposed. Care should be taken not to let such a situation arise and, if need be, to treat the patient with methylene blue intravenously.

12.7   Summary

- Among the irritants, corrosives and caustics are common mineral acids and alkalis, together with some domestic products, e.g. oven cleaners
- On the skin and mucosae these can cause irritation and ulceration. The affected area should be liberally irrigated with water, or saline, and then treated as a thermal burn. For hydrofluoric acid, calcium gluconate should be applied
- Irritants, corrosives and caustics are all damaging to the eyes which, when affected, should be promptly and copiously irrigated and then expert, ophthalmic advice should be sought
- When such substances are swallowed they usually injure the mouth, pharynx, oesophagus and stomach, with vomiting, haematemesis and collapse. The gut may be perforated and, later, it may be the site of scarring and stenosis, necessitating surgical intervention
- Gastric aspiration and lavage should be withheld, and no attempt should be made to neutralise the acidity or alkalinity, but active, supportive treatment should be given
- Sometimes corrosives on the skin can prepare the way for systemic toxicity which may demand specialised treatment

12.0 Irritants, corrosives and caustics

Notes

12.0 Irritants, corrosives and caustics

Notes

12.0   Irritants, corrosives and caustics

Notes

13.0 Household products

13.0 Household products

13.1 Household bleaches / 13.2 Lavatory sanitisers

These embrace a wide variety of chemically based formulations. They have attracted much concern toxicologically, principally owing to the dangers that they are said to constitute for small children, who may innocently handle and swallow them.

13.1 Household bleaches

Domestic hygiene and fastidiousness in the home have created a large market for bleaches, which are mostly solutions containing, essentially, 3-6 % of sodium hypochlorite. On the skin and mucosae, or even in the eyes, this concentration is of comparatively little consequence. In the stomach, however, hypochlorous acid may be formed. The ingestion of relatively small volumes, as with accidents to children, can be dealt with simply by giving water, or better still, milk, as a diluent and demulcent. More active treatment is better withheld, for the toxic consequences are nearly always negligible. Larger volumes imbibed suicidally must be treated in the same manner as for other corrosive acids.

13.2 Lavatory sanitisers and deodorants

These are of different kinds, but the prevailing types contain dichlorobenzene. The amounts nibbled by children seldom cause any trouble, but if larger quantities, i.e. several grams, are actually swallowed, the symptoms evoked may include vomiting, diarrhoea, abdominal pain and, possibly, kidney and liver damage. So where there is reason to believe that, owing to the dosage, this may happen, the stomach should be emptied and treatment should be applied symptomatically as appropriate.

Quite unexpected accidents can nevertheless come about through disregard of the warnings on bleach containers when someone, intent on a high standard of lavatory cleanliness, pours bleach down a toilet pan into which other cleaners, especially those based on bisulphates, have already been introduced. The ensuing chemical reaction may briskly liberate gases such as chlorine, oxides of sulphur, or even chloramine. These are potent, respiratory irritants for which symptomatic treatment must be given at once.

13.0 Household products

13.3 Dishwashing powders and granules

Products of this kind, intended for dish-washing machines, may be irritant, or corrosive. Unless swallowed deliberately and excessively, the quantities taken produce few, if any, symptoms. The stomach need not be emptied and drinks of water, fruit juice, or milk usually suffice by way of treatment. Unsuspected irritation of the oesophagus, or stomach, has nevertheless been described, the more so in children, even when there is no indication of any such reaction in the mouth or throat. Caution, with ongoing observation, is therefore counselled. In case of doubt, endoscopy may be helpful.

13.4 Dishwashing liquids

These are potentially irritant and may be caustic. Yet experience shows that attempts to swallow anything approaching a harmful quantity are frustrated by choking, retching and coughing. Washing-out the mouth and giving simple fluids to drink should afford sufficient relief.

13.5 Household detergents

These are domestically commonplace. Taken by mouth they may cause vomiting. Their clinical toxicity is negligible. Treatment is the same as for dish-washing liquids.

13.6 Disinfectants

The chlorinated phenols and xylols, being the chemicals that have taken the place of phenol in most modern household disinfectants, are of low toxicity. They may, however, be admixed with isopropyl alcohol (propan-2-ol) that, towards the human body, behaves as ethanol, only more powerfully. So if they have been swallowed, the stomach should be emptied and any sequelae should be treated as for ethanol overdose (see **8.15**).

13.0   Household products

13.7   Metal polishes, etc.

Often the vehicle for these products is some sort of petroleum
hydrocarbon. Rarely do they lead to any harm when swallowed
and, as bronchial aspiration is the major hazard, it is better not to
try to empty the stomach, but just to relieve any minor symptoms
that are evident.

13.8   Cosmetics

Taken accidentally by mouth the cosmetics can, in practice,
be virtually disregarded toxicologically. Even when inordinately
large quantities are ingested gastric aspiration and lavage, or
induced emesis, may still be superfluous and treatment should be
limited to palliative measures. Toilet waters, however, with their
large content of ethanol, may be inebriating if drunk in quantities
beyond 50-100 ml.

13.9   Potable liquors

Apart from a few strictly teetotal households and those in which
alcohol is firmly proscribed on religious grounds, there can be few
homes wherein spirits, wine, beer, cider, etc. are entirely out-of-
reach. Overdose, by accident or intent, is therefore, an ever-
present possibility. When this arises the treatment is that for
ethanol poisoning (see **8.15**).

13.10   Kettle descalers

These commonly contain about 40% formic acid and mishaps
with them demand suitable attention as for corrosives (see **12.0**).

13.11   Battery acids

Medically these should be accorded the respect they deserve as
mineral acids, i.e. corrosives (see **12.0**).

13.0   Household products

13.12   Drain cleaners; oven cleaners

Most of these are based on strong solutions of caustic soda. With oven cleaners supplied as aerosols the eye may be especially vulnerable. Treatment of any spillage on the person, or of ingestion, should be as for caustics (see **12.0**).

13.13   Summary

- Most household products on the market nowadays are toxicologically of little concern. Unless swallowed deliberately in excessive quantities, e.g. more than 200-300 ml, they induce little more than retching, a little vomiting and mild, abdominal discomfort
- Active treatment should be avoided, the stomach need not be wilfully emptied and bland drinks should be given as palliatives. Hospital admission is thus superfluous
- The exceptions to this generalisation include phenol (rarely met with today as a disinfectant), kettle descaler (formic acid), drain and oven cleaners (caustic soda, see **12.00**), and paint stripper (methylene chloride). These materials can be particularly hazardous if ingested and call for hospital care, albeit symptomatically
- The presence in the home of unguarded, alcoholic drinks is a toxic temptation to children that should never be condoned

13.0 Household products

Notes

13.0 Household products

Notes

14.0 Poisonous plants

14. Poisonous plants

14.1 Fungi

Throughout the world poisonous plants flourish, both in nature and as cultivated specimens. Pharmacologically active botanical species, moreover, have long been turned to account medically, among which digitalis from the foxglove and atropine from belladonna may be cited. The potential for human calamities from this source would, on the face of it, seem to be enormous. In practice, though, man is a wary creature and the hostages to such misfortune are principally children, who are not so discerning.

In dealing with this problem clinically the physician is confounded on two sides; first, the accurate botanical identification of the particular vegetation involved and, second, the ignorance that continues to surround the toxic principles naturally elaborated, their properties and their potency. Generally, therefore, the management of such emergencies can extend no further than the accepted procedures for resuscitation and symptomatic relief. Rarely are any specific forms of treatment applicable.

Reassuringly, in the so-called 'developed' countries at least, the morbidity and, more especially, the mortality, from plant poisoning has been shown to be of a very low incidence. Recovery is the rule, without menacing symptoms and without intensive or exotic treatment.

Nevertheless, whenever plant poisoning is suspected, the patient deserves all the observation and care that befits anyone thought to be the subject of an unknown toxin, without becoming unduly excited or alarmed in the belief that a biological agent is necessarily more noxious than a chemical substance that has been more toxicologically characterised.

Within these generalisations there may nevertheless be scope for expounding upon a few specimens that are either of inherent toxic interest, or constitute epidemiologically a recognised toxicological problem.

14.1 Fungi

Fungal poisoning may be due to the culinary preparation of toxic species gathered in mistake for edible varieties, or to children naively eating what they believe to be 'mushrooms' growing wild.

14.0 Poisonous plants

14.1 Fungi

Amanita phalloides ('death cap')

Not so much in Britain, but disconcertingly elsewhere in the world, illness and death from eating this fungus are all too frequent, even if the appearance of this 'mushroom' is far from appealing.

The toxins embodied in this species fall into two groups; one that is rapidly acting upon the gut and another that makes a more delayed impact upon the liver and kidneys.

Some hours after ingesting *Amanita phalloides* there are abdominal pains, vomiting and diarrhoea, and these symptoms may be sufficiently violent as to cause collapse through water and electrolyte loss. Then there may be an interval of apparent recovery before the onset of damage to the liver, kidneys, heart and central nervous system, with hepatic necrosis most conspicuous. Occasionally the whole course of events may be rapidly fulminating.

At some centres it is possible to estimate the toxin titre by radioimmunoassay, though this is not an indispensible prerequisite to diagnosis or treatment.

A series of allegedly specific methods of treatment have been vouchsafed, e.g. antiphalloidin serum, but beyond the ranks of the devoted enthusiasts there is no convincing proof of efficacy for any of these remedies. Gastric aspiration-and-lavage, reasonable enough soon after ingestion, is probably pointless once the signs and symptoms have declared themselves. Only an intensive supportive regime can then offer any hope, with haemodialysis for renal failure. There is some belief that early dialysis may remove the toxins before they are irreversibly bound to plasma proteins. And this procedure, coupled with penicillin or sulphamethoxazole, or better still silibiuin by intravenous infusion to displace the toxins, is finding increasing favour. In case of liver failure, the customary regime for this condition must be adopted.

Amanita pantherina ('panther cap')

This fungus may easily be confused visually with similar looking edible species, e.g. the 'tone blusher'. Its toxicity derives from the muscarine-like alkaloids which it contains. Symptoms usually come about within an hour or two of ingestion and are of a 'muscarinic' form, with diarrhoea, cramping abdominal pain, bronchoconstriction, dyspnoea, salivation and hallucinations. These may go on to total collapse.

There is no confirmatory diagnostic test. Except when vomiting has already been profuse, the stomach should be emptied by emesis or lavage. Atropine should then be given by injection to reverse the muscarinic effects, though more cautiously than with organophosphate pesticide poisoning, for it happens that the *A. pantherina* toxins can themselves exhibit atropine-like actions and, besides this, disorientation and hallucinations may become intensified.

Amanita muscaria ('fly agaric')

In contradiction to its botanically specific name this fungus is virtually free from muscarine. The symptoms are largely hallucinatory and they are best controlled by chlorpromazine, or a similar drug. This fungus is subject to deliberate abuse for its psychotomimetic effects.

Psylocybe semilanceata ('liberty cap') and *Panaeolus foenisecii*

These species, like *Amanita muscaria*, are mainly hallucinogenic, a property upon which members of deviant cultures, or movements, have seized upon in their quest for unworldly and escapist forays. People so indulging may be misdiagnosed as suffering from an alcoholic excess, with wildness and aggression. Treatment is by restraint, sedation and tranquillisation, to which end chlorpromazine may be helpful.

Coprinus atramentarius ('ink cap')

This small, dark-coloured fungus, which grows exuberantly and is often seen in domestic grasslands and lawns, is not directly toxic. Instead, it possesses a disulfiram (Antabuse)-like action, by virtue of a constituent that behaves as an alcohol dehydrogenase inhibitor. So, when it is eaten and an alcoholic drink is taken subsequently, it gives rise to flushing, dyspnoea, throbbing headache, palpitation and vomiting, often to a terrifying degree.

14.0 Poisonous plants

14.1 Fungi

Other plants

A catalogue of all the plants in Britain thought to be poisonous
would expand to a volume in itself. Such texts have been published. A complete list of the toxic flora throughout the world
would be extensive indeed. Even so, the toxic principles which
they harbour remain largely unexplored and their attribution is too
often limited to a designation that is no more than a manipulation
of the botanical name, e.g. oenanthotoxin from *Oenanthe
crocata*, the Hemlock Water Dropwort. More exact, physical,
chemical and toxicological characterisation and, critically, quantitative potency, is a largely unexplored area.

This ignorance is enough to strike the terror of incompetence into
any physician looking after a patient supposed to have been
poisoned by some plant or another. To begin with, he may well
be unable to identify the supposedly offending vegetation. He will
have no idea about its toxic content. He is unlikely to have any
reliable indication of the dose ingested. So what can he do?
Maybe a poisons information centre can grant him a little enlightenment (Appendix 1). What in the end, though, will confer solace
upon him, is the realisation that irrespective of all these considerations, the treatment is universally the same—symptomatic and
supportive.

The clinical signs may be neither pathognomonic, nor diagnostic.
Nausea, vomiting, diarrhoea, along with some abdominal pain,
are well-nigh invariable, to a lesser or greater degree. There may
also be dyspnoea, weakness, paraesthesia, neuropathy and
sometimes convulsions; at other times restlessness, excitement,
visual disturbances and hallucinations. Seldom is there coma.

Laboratory tests are out of the question, except in the odd cases
when investigations are conducted later for forensic purposes.
And where a patient is in the throes of respiratory depression, or
convulsive seizures, to pore over a pictorial chart in the search for
botanical identification is tantamount to culpable waywardness.
As already emphasised, the principles of treatment are the same,
whatever the aetiology. If the evidence points to a substantial
amount of some plant, leaf, berry, root, etc., having been eaten
within the last 4-6 hours and spontaneous vomiting has not
already taken place, then the stomach should be emptied, if only
as a precaution, by induced emesis, or by gastric aspiration and

14.0 Poisonous plants

14.1 Fungi

lavage. Thereafter, unremitting observation should be continued for at least 24 hours. Fluid and electrolyte balance should not be allowed to become disordered owing to, say, vomiting and diarrhoea, but any deficits should be made good. Ventilatory assistance should be provided if respiration becomes embarrassed. Convulsions should be controlled by diazepam injections and excitement, hallucinations, etc., should be controlled by giving chlorpromazine, or such-like drug.

Careful collation of case-histories covering large numbers of patients, most of them children supposedly poisoned by plants, has revealed that adherence to these supportive and symptomatic modes of treatment has been enough to ensure early and total recovery almost without exception.

14.0 Poisonous plants

Notes

14.0 Poisonous plants

Notes

14.0 Poisonous plants

Notes

15.0 Animal poisons

15.0 Animal poisons

15.1 Venomous snakes

Outstanding among the toxicologically offensive animals are the poisonous snakes, although there are many other creatures equally capable of delivering dangerous bites and stings. The haunts of the various species coming into this category, although they are spread around the world, are nevertheless irregularly dispersed and it behoves the physician to be acquainted with the venomous fauna in the neighbourhood in which he practises, so as to be prepared for any emergency emanating therefrom.

15.1 Venomous snakes

In Britain there is only one native poisonous snake, *Vipera berus* (the common adder), but the possibility always exists of more exotic and vicious specimens escaping from public zoos or, more so, from private hands. This notwithstanding, the incidence and severity of snake bites in Britain give no grounds for anxiety.

In other parts of the world much more lethal species flourish, the wilder territories being their chosen haven. In some areas casualties and deaths from snake bites are believed to reach enormous proportions, even if there are no dependable epidemiological statistics to support this opinion.

The true vipers (*Viperinae*) are located all over the world, except for America and the Asian and Pacific regions, whereas the pit vipers (*Crotalidae*), including the rattlesnake, are encountered in Asia and America. The cobras, mambas, etc. (*Elapidae*) have world-wide habitats, apart from Europe. Only in Asian and Pacific waters do sea snakes abound.

Bites are usually inflicted upon the limbs, because of their proximity to the snake, and rarely upon the trunk or head. The venom may be localised to the site at which it is introduced, generating only local reactions, or it may spread, first to the neighbouring lymph nodes and then, maybe within an hour or so, to other tissues of the body, continuing thus to circulate for a considerable time.

Action

The venom of both the true and pit vipers is principally vasculotoxic and, while the distinction is by no means rigid, that of the *Elapidae* is more necrotising and neurotoxic, with neuromuscular blockade. Sea-snake venom is predominantly myotoxic.

15.0 Animal poisons

15.1 Venomous snakes

Signs and symptoms

These will depend ultimately on the particular snake responsible and the victim may be able to recognise this for himself. Understandably the creature is seldom captured for identification. That is why the physician should be aware of the likely venomous assailants within his realm.

Snake-bite is not synonymous with envenomation and it is claimed that about half the number of people bitten suffer no ill-effects, because the venom has not actually been injected through the skin. Puncture marks are nearly always visible and, with envenomation, swelling, pain and necrosis may be obvious within half-an-hour.

Systemic shock may quickly encompass the patient, with vomiting, diarrhoea and collapse. This stage may resolve on its own, but not invariably. Shock of later onset is of more ominous portent. Then there may be devastating collapse, with cardiac dysfunction, and sometimes pulmonary oedema.

The other complications are related to the type of snake responsible. With the true vipers and the pit vipers there is haemo-concentration, thrombocytopenia, interference with blood clotting, intravascular coagulation and spontaneous haemorrhage. Acute renal failure may be concomitant.

With the *Elapidae* the local reaction is less marked and the muscular weakness is seen first in the eyes, tongue and throat, with ptosis and dysphagia. This is succeeded by more widespread neuropathy, with respiratory failure as the chest becomes involved.

With the *Hydrophidae*, or sea snakes, generalised myopathy can be seen after a lapse of some hours, with depressed tendon reflexes and, later, myocardial failure. There may also be myoglobinaemia and renal failure.

Diagnosis

This must, of necessity, be largely circumstantial and there is no laboratory test that is of any assistance.

Treatment

History and local practice is replete with folklore on the treatment

15.0 Animal poisons

15.1 Venomous snakes

of snake bites: most of it, if not positively exacerbating, is at least unrewarding. Effective management today relies on two approaches; local measures and sufficient antivenom.

Ideally it should be confirmed whether mere biting has occurred, or whether this has proceeded to actual envenomation. For the inexperienced clinician, this is not easy to decide, though the absence of local swelling within an hour or so is reassuring, while on the other hand generalised symptoms leave no doubt.

First-aid should rely on the application of a pressure bandage at the site of envenomation. This is far preferable to a tourniquet. The former can be left in place for some hours, though neither procedure is feasible, of course, for bites to the neck. No other local intervention, e.g. incision, should be countenanced.

Then, if it is accepted that envenomation has taken place, the proper antivenom should be prepared without delay, for as soon as systemic damage has advanced it cannot be reversed. If this antivenom is not locally to hand, some countries at least conserve supplies for emergency use at strategic centres. The patient is best looked after in a unit with intensive care facilities, so that oxygen, airways, suction apparatus, etc., are within reach.

Anxiety and panic can easily assail the patient, who should therefore be sedated with diazepam. Morphine is better withheld.

For the antivenom, preliminary skin testing for sensitivity is as unnecessary as it is uninformative, but adrenaline should be injected subcutaneously as premedication, and a dose of a systemic corticosteroid should be administered to anyone known to be, or thought to be, allergic, or who is said to have received horse serum previously. Care should be taken to see that the antivenom is not at all opaque, for this implies loss of potency, and if a freeze-dried preparation is difficult to dissolve, then a suitable, sterile filter should be set up in the intravenous line.

The antivenom is conveniently mixed with Hartmann's solution, one-in-ten by volume, and infused intravenously at the rate, to start with, of about 15 drops per minute. At the first sign of an adverse reaction the drip should be stopped and the premedication should be repeated before restarting. This expedient may have to be replicated two or three times before the infusion can carry on uneventfully. Thereafter the rate may be advanced, with the intention of completing the instillation of the first antivenom dose within about an hour. If the patient's response should not be favourable enough, further infusions should be undertaken, up to as many as 10 ampoules in all.

The usual supportive measures should be actively applied meanwhile to counteract shock and to overcome fluid and electrolyte depletion, especially that of potassium, for hypokalaemia is often severe in myotoxic envenomation. The pulse, blood pressure, fluid balance, electrocardiogram, blood picture and blood urea should all be monitored. As soon as the venom has been adequately neutralised, any coagulation defects should be rectified specifically, or by transfusions of fresh blood, but heparin should not be given.

Locally the wound can be infected. Anti-tetanus prophylaxis is obligatory and antibiotics may be required. Heroic, surgical assaults locally should be forsworn. Instead, only careful debridement for local necrosis should be permitted.

Throughout, the respiration should be safeguarded and, if renal function should falter, then haemodialysis, or peritoneal dialysis, may have to be brought into action.

No patient with a story of snake-bite should be summarily dismissed without careful examination, and no patient who has emerged successfully from treatment should be discharged until careful observation and investigation have endorsed complete recovery, i.e. usually about a week or so later.

15.2   Bee stings

The honey bee (*Apis mellifera*) stings by impelling a venom gland, surmounted by a barb, into its victim. Through this apparatus the alkaline venom is injected locally into the tissues, causing inflammation around the site. The sting barb should be removed as soon as possible from the skin, not by forceps, but by scraping it off, preferably by the blade of a knife. Then the application of a mild acid, such as vinegar, is said to be soothing.

Multiple stings can sometimes prove serious and any that are in the vicinity of the mouth or pharynx can, by the swelling that develops, embarrass the airway and put the patient in danger.

Besides any local measures, then, an attempt should be made to overcome the oedema by a systemic injection of adrenaline, by mechanically establishing an airway, or in extreme cases by tracheostomy.

The more far-reaching reactions generally arise, however, because the person is already sensitised, for then the sequelae may be disastrous, again when the oedema extends critically to the throat and larynx. At this juncture, immediate injections of adrenaline intramuscularly may be life-saving. Alternatively and in less extreme cases, adrenaline inhalations, or antihistamines parenterally, may be given. Corticosteroids may also be remedial.

Those people known to be sensitised should be at pains to keep clear of bees. They can also be protected by a course of immunotherapy with whole bee venom injections over a period of 20 weeks.

15.3 Wasp, hornet, and etc. stings

These present similar problems to the stings of bees and should be managed therapeutically along just the same lines. Immunotherapy is not practicable. The fire ant (*Solenopsis xyloni*) can set up remarkably severe anaphylactic reactions, either at once or later on, and these demand very prompt anti-allergic medication, primarily with injections of adrenaline and then, possibly, with corticosteroids.

15.4 Scorpions

Where scorpions (*Centruroides*) loiter in human surroundings, usually in the tropics and sub-tropics, they can become a menace. Their stings cause intense, local pain, while general sweating and hyperparaesthesia develop, sometimes progressing to respiratory and cardiac depression.

Direct immobilisation by a pressure pad is the primary remedy, with the customary supportive management for systemic complications. Supplies of antivenom are said to be procurable in Mexico City alone.

15.5   Spiders

However distasteful their appearance, the spiders at home in temperate climates are not hostile to man, whereas some of those lurking in the warmer regions are far from amicable.

The female, but not the male, of the Black Widow Spider (*Hactrodectus mactans*) executes a bite that, after a few minutes, becomes excruciatingly painful locally. Next there is tender, regional lymphadenopathy and, after a few hours, there may be headache, vomiting, pain in the abdomen and in the limbs, pyrexia, muscle spasms and a raised blood pressure.

The wound should be cleaned, but local pressure should be withheld, cooling dressings should be applied, analgesics administered for the pain and supportive measures provided as required. Patients severely affected should be given the specific antivenom intramuscularly or intravenously, if it can be obtained.

Spiders of the genus *Loxosceles*, notably the Brown Recluse Spider (*L. reclusa*) are to be found in the southern parts of America, more so in the summer than in the winter. Their bites may at first go unnoticed. Then the victim becomes aware of acute pain locally, with inflammation and blistering in the area. This zone tends to spread widely, with haemorrhagic necrosis. Systemically there may be pyrexia and vomiting, with a spreading, itchy, morbilliform rash and, in a few cases, haemolytic anaemia, thrombosis and jaundice. Deaths are recorded.

Diagnostically this condition must be distinguished from anthrax, erysipelas, dermal burns and in, advanced cases, *Clostridium perfringens* infection. Treatment is directed to local cleansing and pressure dressings, with general supportive measures and antibiotics for secondary infection. Delicate debridement may encourage healing and, later, if the scarring becomes disfiguring, it may be ameliorated by plastic surgery.

A specific antiserum is said to have been prepared in Peru, but it does not seem to be available elsewhere.

15.6   Venomous fish

Venomous marine creatures are more populous in tropical and

sub-tropical waters than in temperate zones. Their stings hardly ever prove fatal, apart from those of sea snakes (**15.1**).

There are said to be about two hundred species of venomous fish, their bodies being embellished with spines that represent a threat to anyone in contact with them, either by physical injury (e.g. some of the sharks), or by envenomation (e.g. the sting-ray (*Urobatis halleri*), the weever fish (*Trachinus draco* and *Tr. vipera*), the scorpion fish (*Scorpoenidae*) and some catfishes). With the latter group, entry of the spines into the skin of man at once sets up an acute, fiercely-throbbing pain that seems almost unbearable. The spines should be removed and local anaesthetic should be injected to relieve the agony. Then, as the toxin is heat-labile, the affected part of the body should be immersed, or bathed, in water as hot as can be borne, for upwards of an hour. The wounds are liable to be infected, so antibiotics should be given to protect against chronic sepsis. If there are systemic reactions — vomiting, diarrhoea and shock — these should be treated supportively.

15.7 Coelenterates

The troublesome Coelenterates include the jelly fish and, notably, the so-called Portuguese Man-of-War (*Physalia*). When trodden on, or crushed, these creatures inject a venom percutaneously which sets up local pain of a shooting and throbbing nature, with erythema and pruritis. Vomiting, abdominal pain and muscular cramps may also be experienced, along with generalised weakness. Exceptionally these symptoms progress to paralysis, convulsions and delirium, presaging a fatal outcome. Alcohol should never be applied to the site of injury, but domestic vinegar locally inactivates the venom. Treatment for the systemic illness should be symptomatic and supportive.

15.8 Toxic fish (see 15.9-15.12)

Besides those marine species that in the live state can be hostile, there are a number of fish the flesh of which is toxic to man; intrinsically so, or because of deterioration biochemically after landing, or because they have themselves ingested some other poisonous denizen of their watery environment. The most important members of these three classes are the Cignatera (**15.9**), Tetraodontidae (**15.10**) and Scombroidae (**15.11**).

15.9 Cignatera

When it is remembered that fish make up the diet of so many
members of the human race and, indeed, may be the principal
source of protein for certain large ethnic groups, it is perhaps
astonishing how comparatively little poisoning comes about in
this way, the more so as hundreds of species are claimed to
elaborate cignatoxin in their bodies. This characteristic varies not
only according to species, but also in relation to their habitat,
though the red snapper and the barracuda, as found around the
Pacific Islands, have a bad reputation in this respect.

Action

Cignatoxin is a lipid-soluble and heat-stable compound, which has
been shown to inhibit cholinesterase. Its toxicity, however,
cannot be explained by this mechanism alone.

Signs and symptoms

After consuming cignatoxin-contaminated fish the onset of symptoms may be immediate, or postponed for as long as a day after-
wards. Then there is tingling of the lips, throat and tongue, along
with numbness, and subsequently vomiting, diarrhoea and colicky
abdominal pains. The muscles and joints may become painful,
visual aberrations are suffered and convulsions distress the
patient. Respiratory paralysis may bring about death, which is the
fate of up to 10% of those affected.

Diagnosis

This depends entirely on the history, symptoms and signs.

Treatment

Since treatment can do no more than alleviate symptoms, prevention becomes critical in mitigating this disease. The viscera
of tropical fish should always be rejected for culinary use. Soak-
ing the flesh in water for some days before preparation and
discarding the water is said to dilute the toxin.

As part of the symptomatic treatment, atropine can be helpful.

15.10 Tetraodontidae

Many species of Tetraodontidae (e.g. Puffer fish) form tetrado-toxin (fugu poison) in their tissues, chiefly in the viscera and, to a greater extent, in the gonads. Unfortunately 'puffer fish' are rated as a culinary delicacy in some countries, especially Japan, and there, personnel are expertly trained to prepare the fish for the table, removing the tainted organs. Casualties, nevertheless, still occur.

Action

The selected site of action of tetrodotoxin is the nervous system, more peripherally than centrally. There may also be some effect directly on the muscles.

Signs and symptoms

These appear quite soon after the toxic fish is eaten, with the onset of paraesthesia orally and peripherally, muscle weakness, proprioceptive impairment, diarrhoea, convulsions and respiratory depressions. Death comes about by respiratory arrest and the mortality rate is above 50%.

Diagnosis

The history and clinical features leave little room for doubt.

Treatment

No specific treatment has been evoked, so only symptomatic relief can be afforded, with active respiratory support.

15.11 Scombroidae

Numbered among the scombroid fish are such popular edible varieties as the mackerel, tuna, bonito and skipjack. Normally and in the fresh state they are perfectly acceptable as food, but if they are allowed to spoil after landing, histamine (or a histamine-like substance) is produced enzymatically in the flesh, probably by bacteria.

Action

Scombrotoxin behaves like histamine.

Signs and symptoms

Shortly after eating the tainted fish the consumer suffers flushing of the face, with throbbing headaches, dizziness, a hot choking sensation in the mouth and throat, vomiting, diarrhoea and abdominal pain. The prognosis is good and total recovery can be confidently predicted within a few hours.

Diagnosis

The characteristic symptoms after eating scombroid fish are convincingly diagnostic and almost everyone who has partaken of the same meal will usually have been afflicted.

Samples of the same batch of fish will show, on chemical analysis, a higher than usual concentration of a histamine-like substance.

Treatment

As the toxic attack is self-limiting, symptomatic relief, probably with anti-histamines, is all that is demanded.

15.12   Saxitonin (shell-fish poisoning; 'red tide')

Some of the dinoflagellates which flourish as marine plankton, e.g. *Gonyaulax* spp. and *Gymnodimium brevis*, have the capacity to produce toxins, so that when they are devoured by larger fauna in the sea, either the predators may be killed (forming the so-called 'red tide') or, as with some of the molluscs (mussels, oysters, etc.), they may survive, although the toxin has been imparted to them. It is when these toxin-bearing molluscs are eaten by man that he becomes the victim of 'shell-fish poisoning'.

Signs and symptoms

The syndrome seen after someone has eaten molluscs containing

15.0 Animal poisons

15.12 Saxitonin

Gonyaulax toxin is very similar to that from tetradotoxin and the disease is termed 'paralytic shell-fish poisoning'.

On the other hand, shellfish bearing the *Gymnodimium* toxin have a milder effect and the symptoms comprise paraesthesia, with an anomaly of cold and hot sensations, diarrhoea, vomiting and ataxia—'neurotoxic shell-fish poisoning'. This disorder passes off in a few hours.

Diagnosis

This is based on a disclosure of the eating habits, combined with the clinical presentation.

Treatment

That for paralytic shellfish poisoning is the same as that for tetra-dotoxin (see **15.10**), while that for neurotoxic shell-fish poisoning is simply to relieve the symptoms until they naturally subside.

15.0 Animal poisons

Notes

15.0 Animal poisons

Notes

15.0 Animal poisons

Notes

16.0 Social aspects

16.0 Social aspects

16.1 Child poisoning

Every disease, whatever its aetiology, has some social connotation, for the person afflicted cannot be viewed in isolation. Nowhere is this more impressive than in the realm of poisoning. In an ideal society it should be possible, by modifying the circumstances, be they homicidal, suicidal, or accidental, to prevent poisoning altogether. Even if this should prove a fanciful concept, the physician, preoccupied with diagnosing and treating the individual patient, should nevertheless pay some heed to these wider issues.

16.1 Child poisoning (see also 16.5)

Child poisoning, usually regarded as accidental, in fact arises from a combination of wilfulness and innocence of the consequences. Principally between the ages of 1 and 3 years the youngster proceeds through what Freud called the 'phase of oral development', when it becomes ambulant, explores its surroundings and puts into its mouth almost anything within reach. In most instances this act is inconsequential. It is only when the object or material happens to be toxic that poisoning ensues. In general, children have emerged from this stage of their behaviour by the time they are about 5 years old and after that age, child poisoning is rare, unless they retain the abnormal habit of 'pica'.

In the cause of prevention, any attempt to curb the child's curiosity would be unnatural. Instead, it must be taught discrimination, at the same time as the more dangerous substances are kept out of harm's way. In the ordinary course of running a home it is impossible to secure everything under lock-and-key, but all medicines should be regarded as deadly and kept preferably in child-resistant containers and stored in locked cupboards. Similar safeguards should be extended to those household products recognised as hazardous — drain-cleaners, kettle descalers, turpentine, anti-freeze and so on. The majority of household requisites, on the other hand, are toxicologically insignificant and there is no reason for trying to manage the home as though it were an isolation unit. Nevertheless, once an event of child poisoning has come to notice, it is prudent for someone such as a social worker to visit the home, view the scene and advise on precautions to avoid a recurrence.

16.2 Adult self-poisoning

A relatively large proportion of the population, notably in western society, seems to be encompassed by misery and mental depression. There is an understandable urge to escape from this plight and self-poisoning offers a convenient way out, either temporarily or permanently. Clearly these unfortunate souls are mentally disturbed, though few of them are the subjects of frank mental disease so as to qualify for admission, voluntarily or under an order, to a psychiatric unit. The practice has been to accord each of these patients a psychiatric interview, followed by appropriate guidance, regardless of the severity of their poisoning physically. Unfortunately, this type of support has not been sufficient in itself to deter these people from repeating the act of self-immolation, which may become almost a habit. More fundamentally, their whole social environment calls for modification — a course of remedial action beyond the capacity of the physician. These limitations notwithstanding, the doctor has more responsibility for the self-poisoned patient than merely to overcome the acute stage of the physical illness.

16.3 Accidental poisoning of adults

Official statistics may tend to present a distorted classification of poisoning, with exaggerated prominence being given to accidents. Close enquiry into individual incidents reveals that the drinking, or eating, quite unawaredly, of something toxic is remarkably rare. Carbon monoxide, though, still takes its toll and constitutes the commonest cause of truly accidental poisoning among adults in the home.

Toxic risks to health nevertheless exist occupationally and these are chiefly by inhalation, with percutaneous uptake as the second important portal of entry. Avoidance largely depends, of course, on hygiene and protection, but accidents still arise, by carelessness or ignorance. Accurate diagnosis is important, for poisoning can easily be confused with natural disease. Treatment follows the principles already outlined in this book. Thereafter, the whole circumstances should be investigated so that action may be taken to prevail against any recurrence. Meticulous note-taking is at a premium, for litigation, in which the doctor's records may feature critically, can so often follow. Moreover in many countries there may be statutory obligations to notify occupational poisoning to the authorities.

16.4 Homicidal poisoning

Today, outright murder by poisoning is relatively infrequent, by contrast to previous ages, e.g. those of Nero and the Borgias. This may be on account of the pre-meditation demanded, and the readiness with which detection is effected, apprehension follows and retribution is exacted. Crimes of this kind may nevertheless escape notice unless the physician is alert to the possibilities, retains an enquiring atittude of mind and, given reasonable grounds, is prepared to subordinate that confidence which he owes to his patient to that obligation, which is due from him as a citizen, to the rule of law. Notably this applies in cases of child-abuse by poisoning (see below).

Under British law, the term 'poison' has not been specifically defined. It may be any 'destructing or noxious thing' intended to 'aggrieve, injure or annoy'. Indeed, for the process of trial, the agent may be comparatively innocuous, yet the evil intent, or what is called in legal parlance, *mens rea*, may count against the accused.

Doctors called in evidence for court hearings in relation to poisons should confine themselves strictly to the medical aspects and, if they are dealing with a particular patient, should have made sure that clear and adequate records were made at the time of inter-view and examination—not in retrospect.

16.5 Deliberate child-poisoning

A variant of physical child abuse ('baby battering') is deliberate child poisoning, usually, but not invariably, by means of a drug. Aetiologically this phenomenon falls into one of two classes: first, the child is fractious and keeps everyone awake at night. When it fails to be sedated by the recommended dose of whatever the doctor prescribes, an overdose is administered in desperation, sometimes with dire effects. Then there is the parent, or child minder, who wilfully plies the child with something to harm it. The clinical picture arousing suspicion is that of an ill youngster, baffling the diagnostician, with recovery in hospital and relapse on return home. An exhaustive analytical screening of the blood and/or urine may be revealing in this type of case.

Foremost the doctor must see that the victim is withdrawn and protected from further toxicological assaults. Then the social worker, or social psychologist, or other community services, should be called in aid. A constructive approach in this manner is preferable to police action, which is a last resort, but may well rule out any reconciliation, or unity of the family, in the future.

16.6 Drug dependence

Drug dependence is a social malaise more than a toxicological illness. From time-to-time the exponents of this deviant behaviour become the unwitting subjects of an acute overdose and therefore need active resuscitative treatment. In other respects, it is not so much the physician that can heal them—if anyone can—as the sociologist and psychiatrist. In monitoring their drugs, whether ill-gotten or prescribed, analytical tests on the urine may be fortifying to the doctor in charge.

16.7 'Glue-sniffing'

What has been called 'glue-sniffing' is another bizarre practice that has been adopted by some individuals, chiefly adolescents, over the past few years. A variety of volatile solvents lend themselves to this practice. They have in common the capacity when inhaled to 'transport' mentally those who so indulge. When a plastic bag is employed as well there is always a likelihood of asphyxia. With some halogenated hydrocarbons, especially, there is also a liability to cardiac dysrhythmias and cardiac arrest. With all of these agents an acute narcotic overdose is always a possibility. Physical crises call for immediate medical resuscitation. Analysis of the blood and/or urine may facilitate detection and diagnosis. Treatment of the condition, which fundamentally is a product of personality, is the task, again, more for the sociologist and psychiatrist than for the physician.

16.8 Prevention of poisoning

To deter people from committing murder by poisoning, the sale and supply of toxic substances must be restricted and the fear of apprehension and punishment must be fostered by effective enforcement of the law. To eliminate poisoning occupationally the toxic properties of the chemicals handled must be assessed in advance, hygienic methods and protective measures must be adhered to and provision made for prompt and adequate treatment before serious illness emerges.

Deliberate self-poisoning among adults may be abated, partly by psychiatric care for those at risk and, more so, by modifications and improvements to their domestic and social milieu. Prevention of child poisoning rests on child-resistant containers for selected toxic substances, chiefly medicines, in the home and on continuing education.

16.9 Forensic implications

Injury, or death, by poisoning is properly regarded as 'unnatural'. In most countries the normal certification of death by the physician caring for the patient cannot then be exercised. Instead, the event must be referred at once to the coroner, medical examiner, or whatever other authority may perform in this capacity. It is then incumbent upon the clinician concerned to furnish a medical report of the circumstances prior to post-mortem examination being performed by a pathologist, this being almost invariably a legal obligation. Only then can the authority properly pronounce upon the 'cause of death', be that accidental, suicidal, homicidal, or not ultimately ascertainable.

Homicide is universally a crime that demands police investigations with the object of bringing the perpetrator to trial. In any such court hearing the physician's report and testimony may be crucial; hence the indispensability of accurate and complete medical records noted at the time.

Suicide, on the other hand, is not necessarily an offence, though this depends upon the statutory and religious principles of the country in which it takes place. Once more, though, the findings of the physician may be required for any subsequent official enquiry.

Again, with death from accidental poisoning, not only is the medical evidence required officially to decide the nature of the event but, in many territories, civil litigation may ensue, in the course of which the medical findings may be invoked.

In this connection any toxicological analyses made before death may be of great significance and, equally, any specimens, as of urine, blood and vomitus, that have been obtained whilst the patient was still alive may prove invaluable for retrospective chemical analyses, provided that they have been collected in suitable containers, properly labelled with the name, date and time, and have been suitably stored meanwhile so as not to have deteriorated.

Unaccustomed though the majority of doctors may be to appearing in a witness box, this is always a privilege that may sometimes overtake them. Medical evidence may be factual, pertaining to what was observed or determined about the poisoned patient prior to death (or, for the pathologist, after death), or it may be called for independently, as an expert opinion to assist the court or tribunal in coming to a correct conclusion. In either respect, the doctor should take care to confine his answers to those of medical relevance, within his professional competence and he should never be induced, however persuasive his interrogators, to venture into realms beyond his own, special expertise.

Finally, in dealing with poisoning, as with any other medical disorder, the doctor may sometimes find himself the subject of criticism, leading to the possibility of action being taken against him for his alleged unprofessional conduct or, in civil procedures, for not exercising an adequate duty of care. Wherever this possibility arises no time should be lost in communicating with his own defence organisation, of which he should always be in paid-up membership.

16.0 Social aspects

Notes

16.0 Social aspects

Notes

17.0 Poisons information; poisons control

The last thirty years have witnessed an enormous expansion of poisons information services, or poisons control centres, around the world. Some have come into being by state or official decree, others have been the product of local initiative; many are based upon hospitals, some are apart. They may be staffed medically, or paramedically, and while some may cater for the public at large, others confine their advice to doctors. In essence though, each has the same purpose; namely, to build up an extensive index of items—chemicals, drugs, veterinary medicines, pesticides, household products, and so on—showing their toxicity, the signs and symptoms to which they might give rise, and the treatment that might be applied in the event of ingestions, or exposure by other routes. All aim to answer by telephone throughout the 24-hours. It must be appreciated, though, that all that can be offered is guidance in general, for the centre cannot assume direct clinical responsibility for any particular patient. That must still rest with the doctor, or whoever else is in charge on the scene.

Testimony to the success of these schemes is reflected in the readiness with which their aid is sought and the immense volume of enquiries with which they deal. Any physician will do well to note the address and telephone number of the centre, or service, in proximity to his practice and have no hesitation in making use of it as needed.

There exist national and international associations of these centres and services, for instance in U.S.A., France, Europe, South America and so on, as well as a World Federation. From their membership the list in Appendix 1 has been largely compiled.

17.0 Poisons information

Notes

Appendices

1   Poisons Information Services—poisons control centres

The United Kingdom and the Republic of Ireland are served by a network of officially established Poisons Information Centres providing a 24-hour service for medical practitioners. The addresses and telephone numbers are listed below. On being connected by telephone, the caller should ask for Poisons Information.

London   Poisons Information Service,
New Cross Hospital,
Avonley Road, London SE14 5ER   01-639 4380

Edinburgh   Poisons Information Service,
The Royal Infirmary,
Lauriston Place,
Edinburgh E3   031-229 2477

Belfast   Poisons Information Service,
Royal Victoria Hospital,
Grosvenor Road,
Belfast B12 6BB   0232 40503

Dublin   Poisons Information Service,
Jervis Street Hospital,
Dublin 1   0001 745588

Cardiff   Poisons Information Service,
Ambulance Headquarters,
Old Ty-Bronna,
Fairwater Road,
Fairwater,
Cardiff CF5 3XP   0222 552011

Readers may find it helpful to mark on the above list the centre most conveniently situated for their purpose or, otherwise, to fill in below the address and telephone number of whatever other centre is best suited to their needs:

Address   **Telephone number**

Appendices

1 Poisons Information Services—poisons control centres

People elsewhere who are not already conversant with such a service in their area may seek advice from:

World Federation of Poisons Centres,
Secretariat: Centre International de Recherche sur le Cancer,
150 Cours Albert-Thomas,
69372 Lyon Cedex 2, France

European Association of Poison Control Centres,
Secretary Dr Elsa Wickstrom,
National Poisons Information Centre,
PO Box 1057,
Blindern,
Oslo 3.
Norway

United States National Clearing House for Poisons Control Centers,
US Department of Health and Human Services,
Food & Drug Administration,
Bureau of Drugs—Division of Poison Control,
Room 1346, 5600 Fishers Lane,
Rockville, Maryland 20857, USA

2 Drugs, antidotes and items of equipment usefully to hand for the emergency treatment of poisoning

Emetic. Syrup of Ipecacuanha; Ipecacuanha Paediatric Emetic Draught (BPC)

Demulcents. Liquid Paraffin; Milk.

Adsorbents. Fuller's Earth 30% Sterilised Oral Suspension (for ingested paraquat); Activated Charcoal, e.g. Medicoal (Lundbeck); Sodium Thiosulphate Oral Solution—2.5% (for ingestion of bleach).

Sedatives, Anticonvulsants. Diazepam tablets and injection; Chlorpromazine tablets and injection.

Specific treatments, Antidotes. Atropine Sulphate Injection BP (for organophosphate poisoning/treatment of bradycardia); Calcium Gluconate Injection BP (for ingestion of oxalic acid);

Appendices

2   Drugs, antidotes and items of equipment usefully to hand for the emergency treatment of poisoning

Dimercaprol Injection BP (for heavy metal poisoning); Naloxone Injection 0.4 mg (for opiate overdose); Physostigmine Salicylate Injection 1 mg in 1 ml (for tricyclic antidepressant overdose); Sodium Calcium Edetate Injection—Ledclair (Sinclair) and Penicillamine Tablets BP/Capsules 25 mg (for lead poisoning); Methionine Tablets 250 mg; Parvolex (Duncan Flockhart)—N-acetyl cysteine 20% intravenous Solution (for paracetamol poisoning); Cobalt Edetate Injection, e.g. Kelocyanor (Rona) 300 mg in 20 ml (for cyanide poisoning); Amyl Nitrate Vitrellae (BPC)—0.3 ml; Sodium Nitrite Injection 3%; Sodium Thiosulphate Injection 50% (also for cyanide poisoning); Calcium Gluconate Jelly 2.5%—from Industrial Pharmaceutical Services Ltd., Broadheath, Cheshire; Magnesium Oxide Paste (for hydrofluoric acid burns).

Non-specific agents. Isoprenaline Injection—1 mg in 1 ml; Adrenaline Injection—250 mg in 10 ml intravenous; Dopamine Injection Intropin 200 mg in 5 ml; Dobutamine Injection; Dobutrex—Dobutamine Hydrochloride 250 mg in each vial, to be reconstituted with 10 ml water for Injection, or 5% Dextrose Injection, prior to introduction into 500 ml container for intravenous infusion; Pralidoxime; Obidoxime (as available for organophosphate pesticide poisoning), Snake, etc.; Antivenoms—as appropriate.

Equipment. Guedel Airways—sizes 1, 2, 3 & 4; Laryngoscope, with Mackintosh blade (for adults) and straight blade (for infants); Ambu Bag and catheter mount; Oxygen Cylinder, or supply; Endotracheal cuffed tubes (Portex preferably); Paediatric size noncuffed endotracheal tubes; Reliable and powerful suction; Funnel and tube for gastric aspiration and lavage; Facilities for ECG tracing, or monitoring.

Index

Page number prefixed by 't' indicates tabulated material

Index

Index

Index

Index